The No
Diet Diet

The No Diet Diet

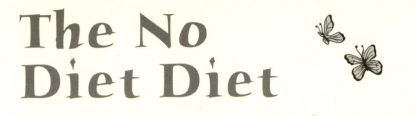

DO SOMETHING DIFFERENT

Professor Ben (C) Fletcher,

Dr Karen Pine and

Dr Danny Penman

Hi JOE,
It's great for boosting creativity
too! The first chapter is a bit hyped-up
but the rest is more scientific.

Danny

First published in trade paperback in Great Britain in 2005 by
Orion Books
an imprint of the Orion Publishing Group Ltd
Orion House, 5 Upper St Martin's Lane,
London WC2H 9EA

An Hachette Livre UK Company

Second edition published in 2007

10 9 8 7 6 5 4 3 2 1

A CIP catalogue record for this book is available
from the British Library.

ISBN: 987 0 75287 400 5

Printed in Great Britain by Clays Ltd, St Ives plc

The Orion Publishing Group's policy is to use papers that are natural,
renewable and recyclable products and made from wood grown in sustainable
forests. The logging and manufacturing processes are expected to conform
to the environmental regulations of the country of origin.

Every effort has been made to ensure that the information in this book is
accurate. The information in this book will be relevant to the majority of people
but may not be applicable in each individual case so it is advised that professional
medical advice is obtained for specific information on personal health matters.
Neither the publisher nor the authors accept any legal responsibility for any
personal injury or other damage or loss arising from the use or misuse of the
information and advice in this book.

Every effort has been made to fulfil requirements with regard to reproducing
copyright material. The author and publisher will be glad to rectify any omissions
at the earliest opportunity.

www.orionbooks.co.uk

About the authors

Professor Ben (C) Fletcher is head of the School of Psychology at the University of Hertfordshire and the founder of FIT Science, which is the basis of the programme in this book. He gained his DPhil from Oxford University.

Dr Karen Pine is a reader in developmental psychology at the University of Hertfordshire. Prior to gaining her PhD, she spent ten years in advertising and marketing.

Dr Danny Penman is a freelance feature writer for the *Daily Mail*. After gaining a PhD in biochemistry, he worked for the *Independent* as a news reporter and the BBC as an investigative journalist.

Between them, the three authors have published more than 100 academic papers and 11 books.

Contents

Foreword by Lorna Houldsworth

Richard & Judy *No Diet Diet* guinea pig

When I appeared on the *Richard & Judy* programme as a guinea pig for the *No Diet Diet*, I didn't realise just how much my life was about to change for the better. Over the first five weeks I lost eight pounds in weight and became immeasurably happier. I didn't have to go on a diet or do loads of exercise. I lost weight simply by changing my daily routines and breaking a collection of habits I didn't even realise I had.

Before I started the Programme outlined in this book, I was piling on the weight at a frightening rate and becoming increasingly unhappy and bored with my life. I was becoming fat and no matter what I did, I just couldn't lose weight permanently. Each day I'd wake up feeling low. I also felt guilty. I had everything I'd always wanted in life: a lovely husband, a fantastic daughter and a delightful house. Despite all this, I wasn't happy. I'd even begun to dislike myself. Deep down I knew I was capable of turning my life around and losing weight, but no matter what I did, I seemed to fail. I just kept on piling on the pounds.

Over the years I'd tried a great many diets but none worked. Each one promised to help me lose huge amounts of weight in record time but every one, without exception, failed me. The *No Diet Diet* is the first weight loss programme I've come across that actually helps you lose weight permanently.

I now realise that most overweight people are stuck in a rut. They are trapped by a network of deeply buried bad habits that imprison them. They often don't know what these habits are because they are so deeply ingrained in the way they think and behave. Until these habits are broken, permanent weight loss will remain just a dream. The *No Diet Diet* helps you break these bad habits effortlessly.

Once I started breaking my bad habits, my appetite naturally declined. I didn't have to diet or consciously cut back on my food at all. This is what I loved most about the *No Diet Diet*: being able to eat whatever I wanted without feeling guilty or deprived in any way. Absolutely nothing is forbidden.

As well as a slimmer body, the *No Diet Diet* has given me a renewed love of life. I used to be a couch potato but now, not only have I lost weight, I've also taken up walking, cycling and skiing. I do regular charity work and I'm about to do a 60-kilometre walk in aid of breast cancer research. I genuinely love doing all of these things. They make me feel better about myself, plus I'm also helping others. Every day I feel happy, contented and much more positive about life. The *No Diet Diet* has given all this to me – and I've also lost weight!

I'll be honest. I didn't expect the *No Diet Diet* to work. Even though it was developed by respected scientists, I simply didn't believe them. I was eventually persuaded by the *Richard & Judy* team to give it a try. I dread to think what my life would be like now if I hadn't tried it.

Please listen to the authors of this book. They have discovered the secret of losing weight. It does work. It worked for me and it can work for you.

Lorna Houldsworth

CHAPTER ONE

Are You Ready to Lose Weight Permanently?

Habits are at first cobwebs, then cables.

Spanish proverb

Turning off the TV, making someone laugh and singing in the bath can all help you lose weight! This book will show you how to eat what you want, when you want *and* still shed around 2lb (1kg) a week.

Sounds impossible, doesn't it? In fact, our scientific research has uncovered the secret of healthy *permanent* weight loss and it really is simple and hassle-free. You hold in your hands a book that is the culmination of many years of scientific research. It explains the secrets of healthy weight loss. But more importantly, our research has unearthed a programme that ensures the weight stays off for good.

The secret of the *No Diet Diet* lies in breaking the old habits that keep you fat. Our scientific research has discovered that overweight people have certain habits in common – and surprising as it seems, it's not overeating. If you break these habits you will lose weight. In fact, we've found that it's almost impossible not to lose weight. What we've discovered is so powerful – and so profound – that it goes way beyond a mere 'diet'. Diets encourage a 'two

> 'I am almost through with the programme from the book and I am very happy to have lost 3.5 kg in 3.5 weeks!' Christa Wolf, Germany

months on, ten months off' attitude to weight loss that leads only to poor health, disillusionment and depression. The *No Diet Diet* leads to permanent, healthy changes in your life and, more importantly, permanent weight loss.

The *No Diet Diet* is different to any weight-loss programme you've ever come across before. If you follow our programme you will lose weight until your body's ideal healthy figure emerges. Then you'll stay that way for as long as you wish. There are no pills, potions or gimmicks. But more importantly, there's no food diet to follow. We're saying forget dieting. Start enjoying life *and* begin losing weight.

The *No Diet Diet* will help you:

- **Lose around 2 lb (1 kg) per week.**

- **Lose weight simply, without calorie or carb counting.**

- **Become healthier, happier and more attractive.**

- **Ensure that the weight loss is permanent.**

This second edition of the *No Diet Diet* is even easier to follow than the first. Our ongoing research aims to make weight loss as simple and easy as possible. This edition takes into account our latest discoveries and also feedback from readers. As a result, we've refined and enhanced the final week of the programme to make it even more effective. We've also fine-tuned other elements of the programme to make them easier to follow.

The diet myth

To understand how the *No Diet Diet* works, you need to understand why diets – all diets – screw up your mind, body and spirit. Then we'll show you how very small changes to your way of life can make big changes to your weight. Our research has discovered the secret of lifelong weight loss. Tiny changes in your life mean big changes in clothing sizes. And what's more, you'll feel healthier, look better, become happier and life will have more meaning.

All conventional diets – and that includes low-carb diets – contain the seeds of their own destruction. It is important to understand that you will never *ever* stay on a diet for more than a few weeks or at best a few months. It is not a question of willpower. Your body has been honed by millions of years of evolution to seek out and consume food. You cannot change this basic biological need any more than you can change your need to breathe or your desire for sex. You will eventually return to normal eating, it is biologically inevitable.

> 'If I lose weight, it all goes back on again when I stop dieting. It makes me very unhappy being fat.' Paula

In practice, this means that when you're on a diet you'll be constantly suffering because:

- *You'll feel hungry most of the time.* If, however, you follow the *No Diet Diet*, your body will naturally tailor its craving for food to closely match its energy and nutritional needs. As a bonus, you'll be too busy enjoying life to feel hungry.

- *On most diets you'll be counting calories, or avoiding carbohydrates, fats or proteins.* In contrast, the *No Diet Diet* is simple, there are no calories to count or carbs to watch.

- *'Faddish' diets lead to unhealthy attitudes towards food.* Our programme helps you re-tune your mind so that you have a more relaxed attitude towards eating. Let us put it this way, if you want a bar of chocolate, just eat it.

- *Most diets encourage your weight to yo-yo.* In fact, there's a huge industry dedicated to selling you diets that don't work in the long run. If they did, why would you pay good money the next time a faddish diet came along? Quite simply, they don't want you to find a diet that works. If you follow the *No Diet Diet* you'll never have to buy a diet book again.

We hate boastful people, which is why we're a little hesitant in shouting out the merits of the *No Diet Diet*. But the diet industry creates so much noise that if we don't clearly spell out the benefits of our programme, then you may never learn about them. So excuse us for a moment while we detail the merits of the *No Diet Diet*. And please remember, it's the culmination of many years of hard scientific research, not the delusions of a big corporation's marketing department.

Five benefits of the *No Diet Diet*

- *You'll lose weight.* Every week you will lose up to 2 lb (1 kg) in weight. That's around 9 lb (4 kg) per month or 2 stone (12 kg) in three months.

- *You will naturally slim down to your ideal weight.* Yes, that's right – the weight that you want to be. In a few weeks you'll definitely be slimmer but, more importantly, you'll be sexier because you'll feel good about the way you look.

- *The weight you lose will stay off.* The secret of dieting lies not in losing weight but in keeping it off. Our scientific research has discovered not only the secret of pain-free weight loss but also the secret of maintaining your ideal weight.

- *You'll be healthier.* Being overweight leads to a plethora of health problems and yo-yo dieting is even worse. If you follow the *No Diet Diet* you will dramatically cut your risks of cancer, heart disease, stroke and a host of other ailments.

- *You'll be happier!* Because the *No Diet Diet* programme focuses on the mind as well as the body, a side effect is greater happiness and contentment. Again, this has been proven in scientific trials of the *No Diet Diet*.

How the *No Diet Diet* works

OK, now you've got this far, we'll tell you the secret of the *No Diet Diet*.

We started our research into dieting because we were stumped: Why were people on diets fat? It may sound obvious: Surely dieters are fat because they are overweight people who want to lose their excess pounds? We realised that too, but we wanted to know the underlying reasons *why* they were fat in the first place. Was it because they ate too much, exercised too little or were they overweight for some other, hitherto unknown, reason? To answer these questions, we started studying the habits of obese people.

At the same time, we did something that was revolutionary: we looked at why people were thin. And we found something remarkable. Fat people and thin people didn't differ so much in how much they ate or exercised but in their *attitude* to the world. Let's put this in context. Haven't you noticed that many slim people (the annoying ones who have it all!) are also the happiest, most carefree and open-minded? You probably assumed that they were happy because they didn't have a weight problem. But have you ever thought that it might be the other way round? That they are their ideal weight because they are happy in themselves? If that was the case, wouldn't it turn the world of dieting upside down?

Let's look at another example. Young people tend to be thinner and also to have a more open and welcoming attitude to the world. Clearly part of the reason is simply because young people

Carol: A typical success story

Is it hard to lose weight on the *No Diet Diet*? Carol doesn't think so. Before beginning the *No Diet Diet*, Carol was around 40 lb (18 kg) overweight. She had difficulty moving around and constantly suffered from aching joints because of all the extra weight she was carrying. Although she was only 32, her doctor had told her that her weight was endangering her health.

Carol had been on numerous diets. Throughout her twenties, Carol would spend May and June each year on a diet, ready for the bikini season and her two-week holiday. She would then spend the rest of the year piling on the pounds. And each year, she'd end up weighing a little more.

'I was a hopeless case,' says Carol. 'No matter what I did, the weight would always creep back. Every diet worked for a month or two, but then I'd start eating normally again. Then I'd get depressed and before I knew it I'd be fat again. Nothing worked in the long run.'

Carol then heard about our research through a mutual friend. We were initially reluctant to allow her on our clinical trial because we were still fine-tuning the *No Diet Diet*. But we relented and were soon shocked by the progress she made.

'After three months I'd lost 21 lb (9 kg)!' says Carol. 'After six months I'd lost 3 stone (19 kg). I'm now my ideal weight and have remained that way for over a year. I can't imagine ever being fat again!'

Carol says that the most important thing about the *No Diet Diet* was that it immediately boosted her confidence and self-esteem.

'But the best thing about the diet is that I love it,' says Carol. 'It's like being a child again. Every day I do something new and exciting. I feel better. I look better. I have so much energy. And, I'm happier!'

haven't had so much time to put on weight. However, it turns out part of the reason is also their open-minded attitude to life in general.

We've found that, by and large, happy, open-minded people have a collection of habits and traits that keep them slim. Obese people, on the other hand, have other habits that ensure that they steadily pile on the weight. We must stress again that the underlying reason is not that these people overeat or fail to go for 8-mile (13 km) runs each day, it's because of their collection of habits and personality traits. To put it bluntly, waistlines expand as habits become ingrained.

At this point you'd be forgiven for despairing a little. 'Oh no!' you cry. 'Not only am I overweight but I'll be forever trapped in a fat body!' Nothing, thankfully, is further from the truth. People are incredibly adaptable. Change is not only possible – it's also quite easy with the programme we've devised (from page 65).

The *No Diet Diet* boils down to this: the more flexible your behaviour is (and the more open-minded you are), the more weight you'll lose. We know this because we've spent over 20 years studying behavioural flexibility in British universities and for the UK Government's Medical Research Council. Yes, we really are saying that if you become more flexible in your daily life you'll lose weight. But not only that, you will be happier, more contented and increasingly successful in all areas of your life.

So what does being flexible actually mean? It means making small progressive changes in your life. Each day you need to do something a little differently. Such things as stopping and noticing things on your way to work rather than rushing to the office.

'The only reason I got involved with the *No Diet Diet* was because I felt I had reached the end of the line. It has been life-enhancing for me ... perhaps even life-changing ... '

Alison, writing in an Internet forum

20 Reasons why the *No Diet Diet* is good for you

1. Weight loss is gradual.

2. Weight loss is permanent.

3. It is scientifically tested and founded on sound psychological principles.

4. It's fun.

5. Relationships are improved.

6. Anxiety and depression are reduced.

7. It leads to a healthier diet.

8. It helps you do the right things more often.

9. It isn't based on restriction or self-denial.

10. It replaces your bad habits with good ones.

11. It opens up new worlds of experience.

12. It deals with the whole person.

13. It starts with your brain, not your stomach.

14. It doesn't focus on food so you don't become obsessed by it or develop an unhealthy attitude towards it.

15. It's a means of grabbing hold of your future, not being a prisoner of the past.

16. It doesn't require drugs, special products or calorie or carb counting.

17. It doesn't disconnect you from your appetite or destroy your natural ability to recognise whether or not you are hungry.

18. It doesn't cause any major organ damage or interfere with your natural bodily functions.

19. It expands your life rather than restricts it.

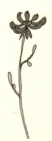

20. It's based on 'Can Do' rather than 'Can't Do'.

It means spending a few moments looking at the flowers in the park, the leaves on the trees, the grip of a baby's hand on your finger, how your loved one looks when they concentrate, the way a musical tune rises and falls, the colour of your friend's eyes, the full moon in a black sky. Yes, all these things really are part of a weight-loss programme!

Being flexible also means subtly altering your character from day to day, or following the whims of your soul. For example, it could mean being more assertive for a day if you're normally too laid-back. Or becoming more passive if you are normally a dynamic, thrusting person. Such things as singing in the bath or cracking an unexpected joke can all help you lose weight.

It all sounds too good to be true, doesn't it? We were once as stunned as you are now, but scientific trials have confirmed that the *No Diet Diet* works. Our promise to you is simply this: 28 days from now you can expect to be around 8 lb (3.5 kg) lighter. You will also be happier and more contented with life. Try it for yourself. You have nothing to lose but your cellulite!

KEY POINTS

- Overweight people have a collection of habits that keep them fat – and surprising as it may seem, overeating isn't one of them. Overeating is a consequence of these habits. Break these deeper habits and you lose weight without calorie or carb counting, hunger pangs or guilt.

- Slim people naturally break the habits that keep other people fat. The *No Diet Diet* helps you adopt these 'secrets of the slim'.

- The *No Diet Diet* is the result of many years of scientific research and has been proven to work in clinical trials.

- If you follow the *No Diet Diet,* our programme will help you to:
  - Lose around 2 lb (1 kg) per week.
  - Lose weight simply, without calorie or carb counting.
  - Become healthier, happier and more attractive.
  - Ensure that the weight loss is permanent.

- You will continue to lose weight long after you've completed the initial 28-step programme.

- There's no diet to follow, which means you'll be more relaxed about food.

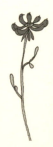

CHAPTER TWO

Be Flexible, Be Slim

**The chains of habit are generally too small
to be felt until they are too strong to be broken.**

Samuel Johnson

Why is it so difficult to lose weight permanently? As an experienced dieter, you are an expert on food, nutrition and exercise. You know all about calories, carbohydrates, fats and proteins. You understand the subtleties of food combining, GI and GL. You also know that, ultimately, the only way to lose weight is to burn up more calories than you consume.

So if you've got all of this information at your fingertips, why don't you just go ahead and lose weight? If only it were that simple! We understand the feeling. No matter how hard you try, you just keep on being dragged backwards. You've lost weight in the past, probably lots of it ... And yet you always seem to pile it back on again. You're fully determined to lose weight. You have the motivation, commitment and

> 'No need to obsess about food or devise a punishing exercise regime'
>
> Independent

willpower to make the necessary changes in your life, and yet you always fall back into the same old ways. Why is it so difficult to make these lifestyle changes stick?

Several years ago, we decided to discover the reasons why the overweight found it so difficult to shed permanently their excess pounds. At the same time, we did something revolutionary, we decided to see how slim people managed to maintain their svelte figures. The results both surprised and delighted us. And when we unveiled them at the annual Health Psychology Conference of the prestigious British Psychological Society, our fellow scientists were equally stunned. Within hours, our work had set off a worldwide media frenzy: we had discovered the secret of dieting screamed the headlines. But better than that, we had discovered the secret of losing weight without even having to go on a diet.

To cut a long story short, the results of our research at the University of Hertfordshire boiled down to this: *you are overweight because you're trapped inside a web of habits that prevent you from losing weight permanently*. It doesn't matter how determined you are to lose weight, if you don't overcome the habits that keep you fat, you will remain forever overweight. *Break these habits, however, and you will effortlessly lose weight.*

'The *No Diet Diet* is better than Atkins'

Sun

We all know that diets work in the very short term but fail in the long run. You can maintain the weight loss for a few weeks, but eventually you 'crack' and return to your normal pattern of eating. Very soon you weigh more than before you started. This happens because all diets fail to tackle the underlying problem of unhealthy habits. And habits govern our lives.

Habit-machines

Habits are natural and incredibly powerful. They help us automate our lives so we can free up our attention and brainpower for other uses. It's amazing how quickly we pick them up. Leave your car or house keys in the same place once or twice and it becomes a habit. Can you remember struggling with your very first pair of shoelaces? Now you can tie them with your eyes closed. Again, it's a habit.

Do you recall how difficult it was to discard the stabilisers on your bike when you were a child? How proud you were when you managed it for the first time? All of the skills needed to balance and ride a bike quickly turned into habits. Even if you haven't ridden a bike in a decade, we can virtually guarantee that you'll still be able to do it. That's how powerful habits are. Once you've learned them, you never forget them. And the more habits we learn, the more we acquire. Our brains are fantastic habit-machines. We can learn something new, and with the speed of thought, it becomes a habit.

As we grow up, our habits master ever more complex tasks. And the older we get, the more we accumulate them, and the more ingrained they become. Do you remember how difficult it was to learn how to drive a car? The mental focus and concentration was immense. Now you don't even notice it. This is the key point: *you no longer notice*. It has become so automatic that you no longer drive, brush your teeth, or tie your shoelaces consciously at all.

> '[The *No Diet Diet* is] the psychological equivalent of the exercise bicycle for the human habit-machine'
>
> Independent

But there's a darker side to habits too. They can also automate and lock in place the things that harm us. Smoking is as much a habit as an addiction. Excessive drinking is too. Habits can also lock in place negative ways of thinking and behaving. Anxiety and even depression can result from habitual ways of thinking. In fact, just about anything damaging it's possible to do to yourself can be locked in place with a habit. If you can think of a way of harming yourself, you can carry on endlessly repeating it as a habit. And again: *you no longer notice that you're doing it!*

The main problem with habits is that they don't exist in isolation. They form a web with other habits. Each one links in with the others, nestling and supporting them. On its own, each habit may not be very strong but, put together, the whole habitweb becomes enormously tough and resilient. When we use the term habitweb we're deliberately comparing it to a spider's web. A spider's web might not sound very tough, but for its size, it's one of the strongest structures known to man. For its weight, spider's silk is five times stronger than steel. It's so tough that scientists are planning to turn it into bulletproof vests. And the way that the spider's silk is woven together makes it incredibly resistant to breakage – just like a habitweb.

Although the whole habitweb may be incredibly tough and resistant to change, individual habits vary enormously in how difficult they are to break. Some are easy to break. You may leave your keys in a certain place out of habit. But you can change that very easily. Just leave them in a different place a few times and you've broken an old habit and created a new one.

The benefits of tackling lifestyle habits

When you tackle your lifestyle habits rather than just your food intake, the benefits are more far reaching too. The people in our studies had to undergo psychological tests at the beginning and end of the trials. We measured their levels of anxiety and depression. After being on our *Do Something Different* programme, they not only lost weight but their levels of anxiety and depression dropped too. This is hardly surprising, because anxiety and depression can be maintained by habitual ways of thinking.

Other habits are more difficult to break. If you're used to driving a certain car and then change it for a different one, it can take weeks to get completely used to it. A few habits are incredibly difficult to change. Eating and exercise habits fall into this category, because they are so deeply ingrained in the habitweb. It's not that the habits in themselves are difficult to break, it's the way that they are supported and reinforced by other habits that determines how resilient they are.

You were brought up to eat a certain way. You spent most of your childhood and adolescence feeding a growing body. In practice, this meant that you locked in place certain eating habits. In the past, these habits would have helped you survive in a world short of food. But in a world crammed to the gunnels with abundance, they make you fat. Eating habits become deeply ingrained inside the habitweb. And they are locked in place by a large number of habits that are equally tough to break.

• 'The roots of your problems lie in the past, but none of the solutions do.'

This is why diets fail. If you go on a diet you are attempting to break your ingrained eating habits by changing the types of food that you eat. But this tackles just a tiny part of your habitweb. You are neglecting all of the other habits that weld them in place. Sooner or later these habits will drag you back. It's not sufficient to tackle just the few habits relating directly to food and exercise. You also have to break those habits that fix them in place. And you can only do this by tackling the ones on the outside of the habitweb. If you do this then the whole web of habits is weakened. As you progressively break more and more habits, day by day, the habitweb loses its grip on you. Very quickly you start to lose weight of your own accord. Your body, once it's stripped of its unhealthy habits, begins moving towards its natural healthy weight.

This is the essence of the *No Diet Diet*. Our programme liberates you from your bad habits. And this means that you lose around 1–2 lb (0.5–1 kg) per week – which is the ideal rate of weight loss recommended by doctors around the world.

As it happens, this is how the slim maintain their ideal weight. Our research discovered that the naturally slim break down their negative habitwebs as quickly as they form. They do this by unconsciously chipping away at their negative habits so that they never imprison them.

So how do the slim constantly keep their habitwebs in check? We discovered that they have a collection of unconscious mental and behavioural tricks that act together to ensure that they're in control of their lives – and not under the thumb of their habits.

In essence, thin people:

1.   **See opportunity where others see barriers and will 'have a go'.**

2.   **Behave in ways that make the most of situations, instead of falling back on their usual old habits.**

3.   **Let things go and move on; they do not bear grudges or rue the past mistakes of themselves or others.**

4.   **Do not make as many references to the past in their thoughts and conversations.**

5.   **Challenge themselves daily.**

6.   **Change their habits regularly and easily.**

7.   **Try new things and experiment.**

8.   **Can be social chameleons when they wish to be.**

9.   **Regularly check out the effects of what they say and do.**

10.   **Have fewer habits and the ones they do have are less fixed.**

Obviously, all slim people do not possess all ten characteristics, but, in general, the more they exhibit, the more likely they are to be thin.

> • Habits breed inertia and inertia is the enemy of weight loss.

We realised that once we understood the secrets of the slim, then we were halfway towards helping the overweight. And this is where the *No Diet Diet* departs radically from any weight-loss programme you've ever tried before. It's based on success. We set out to discover what slim people were doing differently to the overweight. *What they were doing right.* After identifying the secrets of their success, we devised a weight-loss programme that allows the overweight to easily adopt an effortless approach to habit-breaking. The No Diet Diet is the result. But don't just rely on our word for it. Several clinical trials have now been carried out. All have confirmed its remarkable success.

We've also been approached by health professionals from all over the world to help them implement our programme. The message from these professionals is that the *No Diet Diet* can succeed where conventional diets fail.

> '[The *No Diet Diet*] sounds like a sensible strategy. We don't recommend people think about going on a diet, as it suggests that one day you're going to come off the diet.'
>
> Dr Toni Steer of the Medical Research Council Human Nutrition Research Centre in Cambridge

We're obviously flattered by all this attention, but to us the greatest measure of success is the testimonials from successful 'non-dieters'. You'll find many of these throughout this book. And we hope you'll soon join them!

In this book we make no effort to lecture you on eating or exercise. We won't tell you to live off cabbage soup, gorge on fat and starve yourself of toast and pasta. We promise that we won't drive you crazy by banging on about points or calories. Nor will we advise you to stuff yourself with coconuts or agonise over which is the best – GI or GL. We'll simply free you from your habits.

When you are free from these worries, your willpower will cut you loose so that you can achieve what you want. Our research has shown that you will lose around 1–2 lb (0.5–1 kg) per week just by breaking your habits. We have no diet to preach or pills, potions or gimmicks to prescribe. As the newspaper headlines from around the world declared: we have discovered the secret of dieting and it has got nothing to do with food or exercise.

The ten principles of the *No Diet Diet*

1. The human brain is a habit-machine.
It's been fine-tuned by evolution to quickly learn how to do the same things over and over again. Otherwise, everything you did you'd have to learn afresh each time.

2. We're pre-programmed to repeatedly do the same things.
Your brain is equipped with highly sophisticated learning mechanisms. It's very good at detecting subtle environmental cues. The next time you come across these cues your habits drive you to respond in exactly the same way as you did in the past. Have you noticed how often you do things in certain ways, or in particular sequences, even though there's no compelling reason to do so? These might include sitting in the same seat, cleaning the house in the same way, or visiting the same places time and time again. This is partly because one habit leads inexorably to the next and partly because the environment is full of 'hidden' triggers. These can unconsciously send you off like a greyhound after a hare. For example, every night you might go home from work the same way and stop at the same place for a drink or snack. If you went home a different way, these hidden triggers wouldn't crop up, so you probably wouldn't stop to eat and drink.

3. We get trapped inside a web of habits that we endlessly repeat.
Your brain is so efficient a habit-machine that, as you get older, you become more and more habitual. Large chunks of your time can be spent without consciously thinking. You can operate on automatic pilot for much of the day.

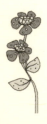

4. Repeating good habits is good for us.

Habits can be good for you too. It means that you don't have to constantly relearn the same things over and over again. It also means that you can use your brainpower for other tasks. Repeating good habits, such as brushing your teeth, is also beneficial.

5. Repeating bad habits means we constantly repeat our past mistakes.

Your brain – like everyone else's – isn't very good at discriminating between good and bad habits. Repeating bad habits harms you physically and psychologically. Endlessly repeating bad habits means you endlessly repeat your past mistakes – no matter how much you try to avoid doing so!

6. To stop repeating our past mistakes we have to Do Something Different.

The power of negative habits is well known to psychologists. Most have tackled them by persuading their clients to try and change their way of thinking. But you can't just change how you think or feel. It's too difficult! Time and time again, research has shown that the best way to break people's habits is to get them to behave differently. It's much easier to make small changes in the things that you do rather than trying to change your whole way of thinking. That's why we start by asking you to *Do Something Different*. If you do something different in your daily life then you'll get something different in return. Small changes build upon each other to have dramatic long-term effects. Very quickly you'll adopt the lifestyles of the slim.

7. The habitweb is incredibly strong.

It's held in place by the forces of inertia, which are far more powerful than the forces of change. That's why habits always beat willpower. If you don't *Do Something Different* then the habitweb stays firmly in place.

8. Breaking the habitweb is the key to improving your life.

Breaking the habitweb sets you free to get what you want. If the habitweb is still intact when you try to make a major change, such as starting a diet, it will always hold you back. You may be able to exert your willpower for a few days or weeks, but eventually the habitweb will draw you back into its clutches.

9. Breaking unconnected habits can unravel the habitweb.

One habit is often fixed in place by several others. So you must first fracture the surrounding habits in order to break the ones you want. These 'unconnected' habits often appear to have little in common with the target habits. Yet they have to be broken in order to get to the target habits.

10. Don't be a habit-machine!

Get what you want by breaking the habitweb. Don't do the same things in the same way all of the time. Have an open mind – one that's alive rather than running on autopilot. Set your spirit free so that it's not trapped by habits. Very soon you'll feel happier and healthier. You'll lose weight, have better relation-ships, plus there's a good chance your career will improve too.

Why is behavioural flexibility useful?

- There will be fewer barriers in your life.

- You will make fewer mistakes and be more effective in all that you do.

- You will be able to make more of yourself and achieve your full potential.

- You will feel better about yourself and have higher self-esteem.

- You will find it easier to interact with people and will be able to deal with new situations more easily.

- You will be less resistant to new ideas and more able to do things that are good for you.

- You will have a deeper understanding of other people and why they behave in the ways that they do.

- You will be more capable of seeing things from another person's point of view.

- Your body weight will change to reflect your behavioural flexibility.

KEY POINTS

- You are overweight and unable to shift it because your bad habits are more powerful than your willpower.

- Your bad habits are fixed inside a web of supporting habits known as a habitweb. You have to progressively break these supporting habits to critically weaken the whole habitweb.

- When you do this, your bad lifestyle habits first weaken then break. When you break these habits, you naturally lose weight.

- Food diets tackle only one part of your habitweb, which is the reason they fail. The *No Diet Diet* tackles the entire habitweb and as a result succeeds.

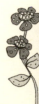

CHAPTER THREE

You are Not a Failure: It's the Diet that Fails You!

Bad habits are like a comfortable bed, easy to get into, but hard to get out of.

Anon.

You wouldn't be reading this book if diets worked. Diets can't, and don't, work. We can't put it any plainer than that. Pause for a moment. If any diet actually performed as promised, then the obesity epidemic would have been cured many years ago. Instead, what have we got? More than two-thirds of the UK adult population are overweight or obese. Even more worryingly, the problem is on the increase. Obesity has grown by over 400 per cent in the last 25 years.[*] At any one time, one in five women in the UK are on a diet; the figure is almost as high among teenage girls. More worryingly, girls as young as

> 'So rapid has been the rise in obesity that there is a danger it will overtake the population to the extent that what used to be considered "overweight" starts to become "normal".'
>
> House of Commons Health Committee Report

---

[*] House of Commons Health Committee Report on Obesity, May 2004.

nine actively consider dieting.[+] And in the US, 45 per cent of women are on a diet on any given day. Does that sound like resounding success to you?

Diets are so ineffective in controlling weight that around

'There is little encouraging evidence to suggest that overweight people generally lose weight; there is ample clear evidence that being overweight greatly increases the risks of a huge range of diseases, and that the more overweight people are, the greater the risks. Yet paradoxically, the phenomenal increase in weight comes at a time when ... there are more gyms than ever, more options presented as "healthy eating", and the Atkins diet dominates the bestseller charts.'

House of Commons Health Committee Report on Obesity, May 2004

95 per cent of people who go on one end up just as fat a year later (and sometimes fatter too). Around half of the people who embark on a diet quit within a few weeks. Every day this is brought home to us when we open our letters and emails. Johanna's letter is typical:

'I'm 39 and have been obese for at least ten years. I am now 17 stone 3 lb (110.4 kg). I've tried every diet under the sun, but none have been a long-term success. On most I managed to lose only 1–2 stone (6–13 kg), but I always seem to end up putting all of the weight back on again, plus more. I've become depressed about my weight and how I consistently fail to shift it. I can see why I should be able to do something about it, but I just don't have the drive to do anything about

[+]   Study conducted by Dr Karen Pine, published in *Clinical Child Psychology and Psychiatry.*

it any more. Being overweight has depressed me throughout my whole adult life. Over the last five years it's got even worse. Everything I've tried has failed. During the last six months I've sought help from my doctor, a specialist and a hypnotherapist. None have helped. You're my last hope.'

Since writing to us, Johanna has enrolled on one of our research programmes. She's been losing weight in a steady, healthy way ever since. She completed the programme in one month as planned and lost 7 lb (3.2 kg) in weight. Five months after completing the *No Diet Diet*, Johanna had lost a further 2 stone (15.5 kg). And guess what? Johanna is still steadily losing weight because of the long-term lifestyle changes made possible by the *No Diet Diet*. She knows that her weight will naturally stabilise around her ideal. If it's a little more, so what? A little less, so much the better. Johanna is no longer obsessed by either her weight or her food. She doesn't suffer from depression, anxiety or guilt. Instead, she focuses on seizing all that life has to offer in the secure knowledge that she's losing weight steadily and healthily.

Johanna – like all of our clients – now realises the reasons why diets have never worked for her, for you, or for practically anyone else.

Dieting fails for many interconnected reasons. Here's just a few:

• **Food deprivation leads to intense cravings, which eventually force you to eat.**

• **Calorie or carb counting – or any other food diet – ensures that you become obsessed with food. If you're constantly battling food cravings, being reminded about food is traumatic to say the least.**

• **Dieting divorces you from your natural feelings of hunger and satiety (fullness).**

- **Diets turn normal food into forbidden fruit – and who can resist that!**

- **Many diets deprive you of key nutrients such as carbohydrates, proteins, fats and calories. This could inflict serious, long-term damage on your body if you don't crack first!**

- **They are often complicated and laborious to follow.**

All diets contain the seeds of their own destruction. Any diet that's based on restriction will fail in the end. This is simply because on a diet, *willpower cannot permanently override the desire to eat.*

> 91 per cent of women recently surveyed on a US college campus had attempted to control their weight through dieting, 22 per cent dieted 'often' or 'always'.
>
> Kurth et al., 1995

A little knowledge of biology and psychology will show you why dieting can never work in the long run. We have all been honed by millions of years of evolution to seek out and consume food. You cannot change this basic biological fact any more than you can walk to the moon. To ensure that we eat enough, nature equipped us with hunger. Trouble is, this drive is distorted by dieting and eventually becomes controlled by a collection of ingrained bad habits. These ensure that 'real' – that is biological – hunger is displaced by 'false hunger'. False hunger is driven by so much more than the natural desire to eat. Habits, emotions, expectations, social conditioning and a wide collection of psychological baggage can all act together to create false hunger. Make no mistake though, if you're on a diet, false hunger feels no different to real hunger. And unfortunately for the dieter, false hunger seems to be triggered far more easily by the outside world rather than the body's need to eat. Pictures of food, the smell of baking and the sight of 'forbidden' luxuries can all trigger false hunger.

If you're on a diet, you control your weight by learning to ignore your body's internal cues, such as biological hunger. You rely instead on external cues, such as the number of 'points' or grams

Dieting depression

On a diet you can become depressed and miserable. Instead of treating yourself with love and respect, you begin despising yourself. One study we ran at the University of Hertfordshire showed the extent to which people who are on a diet suffer from cravings and guilt.

We showed people pictures of chocolatey foods such as cakes, puddings and sweets. We found that the pictures didn't affect the *non-dieters* but the *dieters* experienced powerful cravings and feelings of guilt.

When people are on a diet, these emotions are brought to the fore. Being on a diet makes you crave the foods you are denying yourself. Craving is accompanied by guilt – guilt about desiring something you 'shouldn't' have. Together these all add up to an unpleasant package of negative emotions. The only way you can reduce these negative feelings is by breaking the diet. That brings with it another set of negative emotions and feelings of failure. No wonder dieters tell us they feel miserable a lot of the time. The only way to end this suffering is to stop dieting and find a route to weight loss that doesn't take your mind and body for a ride on the misery roller coaster. And that's what we offer you.

The worst part of this story is that the pictures of chocolatey foods that we showed the people were all taken from diet magazines!

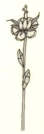

of carbs in a serving of food. In effect, you stop listening to what your body is telling you and instead depend on a book or chart to tell you what to eat. Scientists say that you're 'externalising' your hunger cues. After a while, your brain becomes solely preoccupied with the external cues. Internal ones are ignored. This, in combination with the all too easily triggered false hunger, ensures that dieters constantly walk a tightrope, where one small slip leads to failure.

For persistent dieters, there's an even nastier sting in the tail. When it comes to eating, all of us have an inbuilt 'off switch'. It tells us when we're full and have eaten enough. It's a tiny voice in comparison to the bellowing sounds of hunger. Dieting, it turns out, throttles this little voice, ensuring that you further lose control of your weight.

> 35 per cent of 'normal dieters' progress to pathological dieting. Of those, 20–25 per cent progress to partial or full-syndrome eating disorders.
>
> Shisslak & Crago, 1995

The breakdown in this natural weight-control mechanism has been studied extensively by scientists. Research shows that dieters are more likely than non-dieters to salivate at the sight of food. Or to crave food after merely seeing pictures of it. Other research has shown just how messed up the body's natural weight-control mechanisms have become in the overweight. Most people find food less appealing when they have already eaten. In one scientific study, slim people rated food as less desirable after they had eaten a lot of it. Overweight people didn't. They thought it tasted just as good even when they'd eaten platefuls of it.

Diets sound great in theory, but they all share a major flaw; it's extremely difficult to endure intense food cravings for any length of time. To make matters worse, you are surrounded by temptation. You know that forbidden fruit is the sweetest of all. And to add insult to injury, diets focus on food, which means they constantly remind you about the things you cannot have. If you possess immense willpower you can put up with the cravings

The effects of yo-yo dieting

Years of crash yo-yo dieting can wreak havoc on your body. The actress Britt Ekland has discovered this to her cost. Ten years ago she was diagnosed with osteoporosis, a debilitating condition that weakens the bones, making them far more likely to fracture. Britt is certain that her years of yo-yo dieting are to blame. She recently told the *Daily Mail*:

'I am an actor and staying slim is part of the job, so like most celebrities I have been on a diet for most of my adult life. I would crash-diet for a job and then, when that job was finished, I would allow my weight to go back up again, and then a few months later I would be having to lose weight quickly – typical yo-yo dieting.

'As a result, my body has been deprived of essential vitamins and nutrients, which no doubt contributed to my osteoporosis.'

Now Britt, who on the outside looks just as sprightly as ever, has to take anti-osteoporosis medication to help her bones recover their strength. She says that her experiences should serve as a warning to other dieters.

for a while. But the chances are you won't be able to live like that for the rest of your life. So eventually you'll abandon the diet and go back to your normal way of eating. Once again, your bad habits will have got the better of you.

For a diet to work, then every day – for the rest of your life – will have to be a diet day!

And who wants to spend their life like that? Dieters tell us they wake up in the morning and the first thing they think of is food. Images of toast, chocolate, cakes and chips float through their minds. There's not a lettuce leaf in sight. Through an immense effort of will, these thoughts are pushed aside. This

Forbidden foods

When we conducted an analysis of the number of sweet foods, such as puddings and cakes, that were depicted in magazines we found more of them in so-called 'diet' magazines than ordinary food or health magazines.

Why should this be? It's because the people behind the multi-million-pound slimming industry know what dieters really like to look at – and it's not lettuce leaves! As a result, the magazine editors include articles about how much of these 'forbidden' foods you can have, and accompany them with colourful, mouth-watering photographs.

obviously makes you unhappy. So if you're on a diet, the first thing you feel in the morning is a lingering sense of unhappiness, of paradise lost. It takes a lot of willpower to force yourself to continue living like this for any length of time. The sensual temptations are just too powerful to ignore. How long can you remain in a constant state of self-denial? Is it really possible to be restrained all of the time? Quite simply, no it isn't. We're not designed that way. We are hedonists who will always get our pleasures in the end. And the constant denial is not just miserable, it also induces feelings of anxiety and despair. Not only are these feelings just as corrosive as hunger, they are infinitely more damaging psychologically.

To illustrate the point, in the 1950s, a group of conscientious objectors in America embarked on a controlled hunger strike to see how extreme lack of food affected the human body. In essence, they were starved, studied and brought back to health. The results have been used by relief workers helping the victims of famine and natural disasters ever since. Interestingly, as soon as the conscientious objectors started to lose weight, they became obsessed with food. They spent inordinate amounts of time chatting about food, planning meals and creating recipes. In short, they developed an almost pornographic obsession with food. Sound familiar?

Trying *not* to think about food, when you are famished, is virtually impossible. And thinking about food inevitably leads to one thing – eating it.

Dieting is not a happy state

If you're on a diet, you go through the same emotional roller coaster as the hunger-strikers. Self-righteousness, commitment and idealism all slowly ebb away as the hunger bites deeper into your soul. Unease, anxiety and depression take their place. And as the days pass, you become emotionally and physically weaker, and weaker, and weaker ... The diet inflicts this upon you – it creates a world that is not real and sustains a set of bad habits that will almost certainly make you gain weight in the long run.

After a few days, or weeks, on a diet, the inevitable happens. You have that 'what the hell' moment. That's the time when you decide you've had enough of all the starvation, misery and denial, and give in to temptation. You gladly say 'yes' to the portion of dessert you've been refusing for weeks. You give in, you indulge and, for just one moment, it feels wonderful. Truly awe-inspiringly magnificent. And satisfying too! The thoughts that follow are ones of abandonment, loss of control and guilt. You then think, 'What the hell, I've broken my diet, what does it matter if I have another piece?' So you do. And does that make you feel better? It certainly satisfies your craving for sumptuous foods. But pretty soon afterwards the guilt really kicks in big time.

You feel ashamed because you are now a 'failure'. And perhaps angry too. You feel annoyed with yourself for being so

Why dieting is bad for your mental health

1. Dieting creates an unhealthy and unrealistic relationship with food. This means you will eventually 'crack' and regain the weight you lost.

2. Restricting calories also lowers your energy levels. This can reduce your 'cognitive capacity' or brainpower.

3. Numerous studies link chronic dieting with feelings of depression, low self-esteem and increased stress. Since nobody can stay on a diet permanently you are setting yourself up for failure every time you go on one. Is that the way to feel good about yourself?

4. Believing that being thin will give you more 'worth' as a person reflects the attitude that your self-esteem is dependent on your weight. Dieting doesn't solve self-esteem or emotional problems, in fact, if you get trapped in the cycle of failure, it could make them worse.

5. Dieting disconnects you from your appetite. You don't eat when you are hungry. You then lose the ability to recognise when you are full and should stop eating.

6. By restricting your food intake you may be masking (and thus not dealing with) a more deeply-rooted psychological problem.

7. Any restriction we impose on ourselves leaves us open to guilty feelings. This can lead to depression. Breaking the diet leads to more guilt and the beginning of a vicious cycle of failure.

8. In all but the most extreme diets, weight loss eventually slows down and ceases. This can lead to feelings of despair and hopelessness.

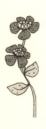

9. Constant calorie counting – and an unhealthy focus on food – can increase the risk of developing eating disorders.

10. Changing your nutritional intake can affect your emotional wellbeing. Dieters often experience mood swings and irritability, which can affect not only them but also their relationships.

'weak'. Angry at the world for making you fat. Then all-consuming disappointment can take over, followed by depression. And you resign yourself to being fat with no prospect of ever being slim. Eventually, the guilt returns – bringing in its wake yet another diet.

Do you see the pattern? Yo-yo dieting leads to permanent unhappiness. It's a habit. A bad habit. You constantly switch from one negative set of emotions to the next in a continuous cycle. If

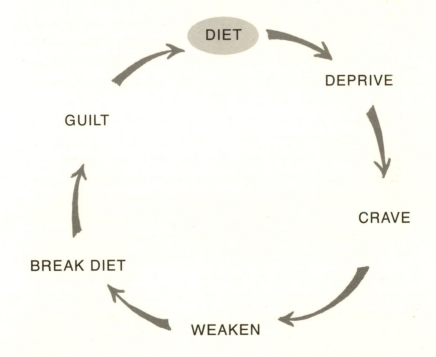

Fig.1 The negative cycle of dieting. You go on a diet. You deprive yourself of certain foods. You start to crave the foods you cannot have. You begin to weaken and give in. You have broken your diet. You feel guilty and ashamed. You start your next diet determined that it will not happen again … but it will!

The illusion of success with low-carb diets

Low-carbohydrate, high-protein diets are supposed to bring about massive weight loss. And for a while they 'succeeded' for many people. People lost lots of weight by cutting out bread, pasta and potatoes. Instead, they tucked into huge steaks and piles of bacon. It seemed to be a miracle diet. But over time people started craving carbohydrates. They dreamed of foods such as toast and pasta until they could resist them no more. And eventually the miracle diet began to look just like any other. That is, it could help people lose weight in the short term but not forever. The cravings eventually became too hard to resist. It doesn't matter which diet people go on, they are all doomed to failure. The very notion of dieting simply goes against the grain of human nature.

you don't break the diet habit you will spend the rest of your life being fat and miserable. Is that what life's about?

The gurus of the diet industry know how to exploit your negative emotions. They understand your depression, guilt and despair. And what do they do? They use your emotions against you. The people who run this industry blame you for the failure of their diets. They say that *you* failed to follow their diet correctly. They never once concede that they're peddling a dodgy product that never stood a chance of working. The truth is: *their diet failed you.*

We constantly receive letters and emails from overweight people. They all contain phrases such as 'I couldn't stick to the diet', 'I gave in to temptation', 'I lost control'. These dieters are far too forgiving. If you're anything like the dieters who write to us, then you should be castigating the creators of the diets that fail to work. You should be congratulating yourself for having the willpower and intelligence to quit the diet habit. You did your best, but it's simply not possible to follow a diet. To lose weight, you'll need to *Do Something Different*. And if all you've been getting in the past is dieting-depression, won't that make a nice change?

The dangers of conventional diets

1. Yo-yo dieting can cause long-term damage to the body's major organs, such as the kidneys, heart, liver and muscles.

2. Constant dieting reduces the levels of the body's natural killer cells. These are vital for fighting off cancer.

3. Dieting can also lead to skin problems, headaches, hair loss, light-headedness, menstrual irregularities, sleepiness, gallstones and constipation.

4. Dieting starves your body of essential nutrients. It's impossible to stay on a diet permanently without damaging your body.

5. Narrow – or 'faddish' – diets ensure that your digestive system becomes unused to certain nutrients. This can lead to digestion problems.

6. Dieting messes up your metabolic rate. Harsh diets slow it and eventually bring about the rebound effect, where even normal food intake makes you even fatter than you were before you went on a diet.

7. Miracle drugs are just as bad and can be dangerous. If in doubt, just read the warnings and disclaimers they come with.

8. Yo-yo dieting damages the skeleton and leads to osteoporosis. Each time you lose weight you also lose bone density. This means that you are far more likely to suffer from broken bones.

9. A single episode of sudden weight loss followed by rapid weight gain can increase the likelihood of you developing heart disease.

10. The production of an important enzyme that encourages the body to lay down fat increases when large amounts of weight are lost. This leads to more fat storage and makes continued weight loss very difficult.

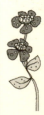

KEY POINTS

● Diets don't work.

● Diets fail you. You don't fail the diet!

● Dieting fails for many interconnected reasons. For example, dieting distorts your natural sense of hunger, which eventually becomes controlled by a collection of ingrained bad habits. This can mean you lose the ability to naturally regulate your own food intake.

● To make matters worse, diets encourage you to become obsessed with food. If you're constantly battling food cravings, being reminded about 'forbidden fruit' ensures that you will eventually give up on the diet.

● Many diets deprive you of key nutrients, such as carbohydrates, proteins, fats and calories. This could inflict serious long-term damage on your body – if you don't crack first.

CHAPTER FOUR

The Science of Doing Something Different

It is not inertia alone that is responsible for human relationships repeating themselves from case to case, indescribably monotonous and unrenewed; it is shyness before any sort of new, unforeseeable experience.

Rainer Maria Rilke

Before you embark on the actual *No Diet Diet* weight-loss programme, we'd like to go into a little more detail about the fundamental principles of the *Do Something Different* approach. This chapter is designed for people who really want to get to grips with the science and psychology behind the *No Diet Diet*. If you just want to lose weight, then you can safely skip this chapter and jump straight to Chapter Five and the start of the *No Diet Diet* programme itself. Having said that, we'd love you to read this chapter and gain a deeper understanding of how and why the *No Diet Diet* works.

Strange as it may seem, the *No Diet Diet* has its roots in 25 years of scientific research into workplace stress and its effects on health. In the 1970s and 1980s, scientists were trying to discover the environmental causes of stress. This soon turned out to be a mammoth exercise, because every time they discovered one cause, another half a dozen appeared.

While working at the Medical Research Council's Social and Applied Psychology Unit, it became apparent to Professor Fletcher that searching for the environmental causes of stress was futile: researchers were simply looking in the wrong place. And many still are. It quickly became apparent to Professor Fletcher that stress came from inside the person and not from the outside world. In most people, it is an internal response to the outside world and isn't generated externally. Most jobs nowadays are not dangerous or psychologically damaging. Compared to the past, we all now have far better working conditions. And today, the things that people in the UK or US find stressful would not even remotely worry a person living in India or Africa. People create stress and, as a consequence, the solution lies in changing the way they interpret their experiences. On a practical level, this means that people can overcome stress by changing themselves and their perceptions of the world, rather than trying to alter the environment in which they live and work. Indeed, stress experts have now shown that changes in the workplace to reduce stress simply do not work in the main. It seems that if you remove one set of problems, another set bubbles to the surface.

A new branch of psychology, known as FIT Science, grew out of these ideas. FIT stands for Framework for Internal Transformation. Professor Fletcher and Bob Stead conceived FIT Science and developed the measuring tools necessary to study it.[*] Briefly, FIT Science is a way of profiling a person's whole psychology. It measures an individual's five key elements of thinking, called the 'constancies', and 15 different aspects of behaviour, known as 'behavioural-dimensions'.

The constancies are, in essence, different ways of thinking. They are: self-responsibility, awareness, conscience, fearlessness and balance. Together they determine a person's 'inner' FITness.

The 15 behavioural-dimensions cover all of the key areas of behaviour exhibited by normal people. For example, Assertive– Unassertive is a behavioural-dimension. It covers a whole

---

[*]   In 2000, they published *(Inner) FITness and The FIT Corporation*, which details the theories behind FIT Science for use as a personal and organisational tool.

spectrum of behaviour from being overly aggressive to complete passivity. Other behavioural-dimensions include: Reactive–Proactive, Definite–Flexible and Risky–Cautious. Taken together, the 15 dimensions govern a person's 'outer' FITness.

According to FIT Science, a combination of these 'inner' and 'outer' FIT elements determine how a person sees him or herself. They also account for how well a person copes with life and gets along with others. Crucially, FIT Science appeared to be a more powerful framework than many other psychological theories for understanding why people think and behave in the ways that they do. But more importantly for us, FIT Science offered people practical ways of improving their lives.

Most traditional tools for change, for example training or therapies, work by trying to get people to alter the way that they think. But this is extremely difficult. Many people simply cannot change the way that they view the world. Another major drawback is their reliance, to varying degrees, on willpower. Many people simply cannot maintain their willpower for long enough to achieve permanent positive change.

FIT Science takes a different approach. Professor Fletcher realised that getting people to change what they actually *do* could be used as a lever to change their way of thinking. Changing a little by *Doing Something Different* gives people a small jolt and sets them thinking along a different track. It can alter the way that they view themselves and, more importantly, it shows them the degree to which they are under the control of their habits.

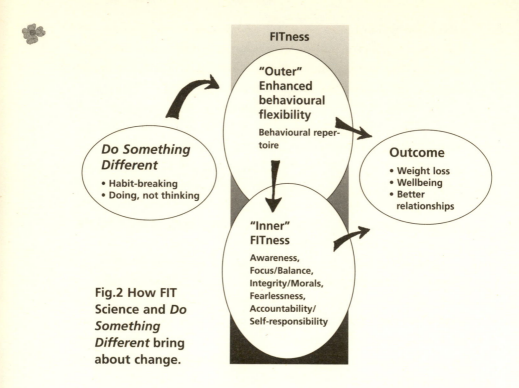

Fig.2 How FIT Science and *Do Something Different* bring about change.

But in the longer term it did more than this. Professor Fletcher found that if people changed their everyday behaviour – so that they became more behaviourally flexible (or adaptable) – then slowly but surely their deeper thought processes began to change too. Often they became more positive, less stressed and generally happier with their life. Interestingly, they didn't need to rely on willpower, the failing of many other 'self-improvement' programmes, counselling and therapies.

So what is behavioural flexibility?

In this context, behavioural flexibility means simply having the ability to choose and then put into practice the most appropriate course of action rather than relying on habit or instinct. It's akin to being adaptable. The more adaptable you are, the more you can alter your behaviour to suit the circumstances in which you find yourself. People with optimal behavioural flexibility are no longer prisoners of their habits.

More specifically behavioural flexibility is:

- **Being able to change behaviour whenever required.**

- **Being able to act after a conscious decision rather than just from habit.**

- **Being willing to try new ways of dealing with situations.**

- **Allowing others to do things their own way.**

- **Expanding behaviours as a means of expanding the mind.**

Crucially, the *Do Something Different* approach doesn't demand that people totally change their personality. The aim is to develop the sides of it that they don't naturally use. The aim is to become more rounded – rather than lop-sided. Behaviour should also be guided by the five constancies, including balance and conscience. The *Do Something Different* approach is designed to help people gain the most from life and not to become self-centred or self-absorbed.

Behavioural flexibility and weight loss

Under Professor Fletcher's supervision, the PhD researcher Jill Hanson began investigating how people's FIT profiles related to their health or, more specifically, their ability to tackle personal projects such as dieting, taking regular exercise and reducing alcohol consumption. It then became apparent from this, and other studies done by Professor Fletcher and his colleagues, that there was a relationship between a person's weight (Body Mass

Index or BMI) and their behavioural flexibility. That is, the less flexible they are, the heavier they are for their height. This was of crucial importance, because it suggested that increasing a person's behavioural flexibility might be an effective way of helping them lose weight. So he then turned his attention to the 'naturally' slim and began studying their behaviour using the tools of FIT Science. It transpired that the slim were significantly more behaviourally flexible than the overweight in certain crucial areas. A programme was then developed to inculcate these types of flexible behaviours into the overweight. It was found that giving people a programme that expanded their behavioural

Health benefits of enhancing behavioural flexibility

Enhancing behavioural flexibility doesn't just improve overall happiness and aid weight loss, it has other, far-reaching health benefits too. Work by Hans J. Eysenck and Ronald Grossarth-Maticek, of the Institute of Psychiatry, University of London, carried out a major set of clinical studies in Heidelberg. They examined the effectiveness of a therapy in which people were asked to create new ways of behaving in situations that caused them unhappiness. The simple changes they made were incredibly successful in reducing subsequent disease and death rates from cancer and heart disease. They also reduced the number of days absent from work and spent in hospital. And, amazingly, the changes prolonged the lives of those already suffering from cancer. Such simple changes improved immune system functioning as well. The importance of *Doing Something Different*, rather than trying to *think* something different, was reinforced by the fact that the psychodynamic therapies had none of these benefits and may even have been harmful.

flexibility led to weight loss. Over the past few years, we have enhanced, refined and optimised this programme to create the *No Diet Diet*.

So why does the *No Diet Diet* work?

For most people (apart from a medical minority) being overweight comes from eating more calories than they use up. This usually makes overweight people think they need to change what they eat. In a sense, this is indisputable – there is no 'magic bullet' for losing weight. Ultimately, you have to change 'the calorie in to calorie out balance'. Nothing, including new obesity drugs such as Rimonabant, can buck this truth in the long term. But that is not where the real problem lies. The problems do not lie in long chains of fatty acids or carbohydrates but in long chains of habits. The reason people are overweight lies not in their food but in the way their poor eating and exercise habits are locked into a negative spiral. And surprising as it may seem, they are fixed in place by a set of habits that have nothing to do with food.

Broadly speaking, there are two types of habit: proximal and distal. Proximal habits are those restricted to just one area of your life, such as brushing your teeth, cleaning the house or riding a bike. These proximal habits are not, as a rule, linked in a chain to other habits and behaviours. When you wash yourself or put on your coat, for example, you quickly carry out these habits and then move on to something else. For most people, these habits are automatic and save time and effort.

Distal habits are very different. They naturally develop much longer chains and do not end with the simple behaviour they started off with but are linked to quite different thoughts and behaviours. Watching the television, for example, is often linked to things such as resting, eating and drinking, as well as many other thinking and behavioural habits. Food and exercise habits fall into this category too. Distal habits have numerous links to other behaviours that appear to have nothing to do with the original habit. They are also more distant from the problem area and usually go unnoticed and untackled.

For example, what you eat for lunch is accompanied by a whole set of expectations, reinforcements, past learning and a social context that is quite independent of the food actually consumed. The food that you eat is a consequence of a large array of connected habits. All of these conspire to make sure that you do things the way you did them in the past. In practice, this means that just doing something as simple as choosing and eating your lunch comes with decades of psychological baggage. Is it any wonder that you find it virtually impossible to lose weight? You simply do not have enough willpower to beat all of these interconnected habits. You will not be aware of most of them and, even if you were, you would not be strong enough to beat the habits of a lifetime.

And this is the central reason why food diets fail. Dieters attempt to lose weight by changing only their food and exercise habits. But according to recent scientific advances, eating is locked in place by a large set of extremely long habit chains – the distal web of habits. It is only when these supporting habits are targeted – as they are in the *Do Something Different* programme – that the dieter can succeed in the longer term.

Endlessly repeating habits

Some people have major problems keeping their habits in check. Obsessive Compulsive Disorder (OCD) occurs when people fail to disengage a habit after they've carried it out. They can build up very long chains of repetitive behaviour. Some sufferers, for example, end up washing their hands many times in a row, or check and re-check their house numerous times to make sure it's locked.

One of the treatments used to help OCD sufferers relies on the Competing Response Theory. Therapists help sufferers break their obsessive habit by providing a 'competing response'. When the person feels a strong urge to perform their habit, they are encouraged to respond with a different, incompatible behaviour. This new behaviour can then take the place of the habitual response, at least until the bad habit has been eradicated. In other words, they have found that an effective way of breaking a compulsive habit is to *Do Something Different*.

While the competing response approach is effective for proximal habits, it has not been applied to breaking the distal habits needed to lose weight. This is another reason why our programme is a major advance.

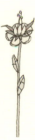

So how does the *Do Something Different* programme help?

Our programme starts with the premise that you have to break down the distal habits in order to lose weight. And we provide you with the keys to change these distal habits by expanding your behavioural flexibility.

Habits are incredibly resilient and powerful. But not only that, many people are effectively governed by their habits. Unsettling as it may sound, habits have a very deep, pervasive control over our entire lives. If this sounds crazy, ask yourself this: Is the average person fully conscious and in control of the way they behave most of the time? Contrary to what you might think, the vast majority of the time, people do things without consciously thinking about them. Why not take a long hard look at yourself? What percentage of your day is *not* consumed by carrying out some sort of habit? The usual range is about zero to 15 per cent. Some serious psychologists suggest the answer is close to zero – at best we have an illusion of control! This means that most people spend somewhere between 85 and 100 per cent of their time being controlled by their habits.

As we've explained, the habitweb is responsible for the majority of your thoughts and actions most of the time. We use the term habitweb because we want to emphasise just how massively interconnected all of your habits are – and how resistant they are to change. This habitweb is made up of both proximal and distal habits. Food diets primarily focus on the proximal habits. Indeed, the whole diet industry seems to be fixated on them. To diet successfully, the industry claims that you have to count calories or monitor arcane units. Or perhaps you have to focus on one kind of food (such as cabbages or coconuts) or limit yourself to low-carb, GI or GL foods. A whole branch of science has been conjured up to dazzle you with its brilliance. Unless you genuinely know your ketosis from your blood sugar, the words serve only to deceive. In a few cases, we do not dispute the science behind the diet. It is true, for example, that a diet high in fat and low in carbohydrate induces ketosis, whereby the body's fat reserves are broken down directly for energy. Low carb diets do force the body to use fat rather than glucose, its normal healthy fuel. What we dispute is whether this is of much practical significance to the person who wants to lose weight in the longer term. Monitoring blood glucose levels is important for the diabetic – but not the dieter.

Of course, some people who go on food diets do manage to lose weight at the beginning. Science does show that such diets *can* succeed, it's just that they tend to fail. Scientific studies show clearly that nearly everyone who diets fails in the end. The science also demonstrates that even when these people do manage to stay on these diets for long periods, their weight loss is not significant. In a comprehensive study of the four main types of food diet, published in the *Journal of the American Medical Association* in 2005, the average weight loss for people put on to the Atkins diet in their trials was 4½ lb (2.1 kg) after 12 months.

Ninety-five per cent of all dieters will regain their lost weight in one to five years. Grodstein, 1996.

But there is another major drawback with all conventional diets: every day is a diet day. The dieter has to exercise willpower *all* of the time. The *Do Something Different* programme does not require this. The habitweb has to be broken or disrupted for the programme to be successful but, once achieved, the

'Although the participants [of the *No Diet Diet*] were not told to improve their diets or exercise more, they chose to do exactly that – without having to apply the willpower needed to persevere with a normal diet. By breaking their usual routine, their fundamental desire to lose weight or be fitter eventually emerged.'

Dr Raj Persaud, *Daily Telegraph*

changes are much easier to maintain because they are self-reinforcing. If the distal habits are changed, the whole habitweb is changed – the food habit-chains are broken and become weaker and weaker, instead of stronger and stronger. Permanent change is much easier with the *No Diet Diet* – and almost impossible with food diets.

If you have any doubts about the rationale behind the *No Diet Diet*, perhaps you might consider a final point. Your personal habitweb is responsible for almost all of your thoughts and behaviours. Food and exercise habits are only a small part of this web. Ask yourself this: Which is likely to be more effective, a programme aimed at the bigger picture, or a food diet that has minor effects on your physiology? Food diets have almost no effect on the habitweb at all. And so you, your habits and your weight will stay more or less the same unless you *Do Something Different*.

If you are serious about losing weight, then changing your habitweb and breaking old habit-chains will begin the process of permanent healthy weight loss. What's more, it will make you feel better about yourself and will give birth to other, more positive changes too. These will make you more successful – and indeed happier – in all that you do.

KEY POINTS

- Weight problems have very little to do with food.

- You are overweight because your habitweb is too strong.

- You may also be overweight because you've been on food diets.

- By focusing solely on food, you are just 'fiddling at the margins' when it comes to trying to lose weight.

- Only by tackling the habitweb directly can you set yourself free and get the weight loss you want.

- If you ignore the habitweb and stick to food diets you are consigned to a life of riding the misery roller coaster (and most of that time as an overweight, unhappy rider).

- Our research discovered a link between one aspect of people's personality – their behavioural flexibility – and their Body Mass Index (BMI). Quite simply, heavier people were less flexible in their behaviours and were more habit-bound.

- We helped people increase their behavioural flexibility by breaking habits and trying new behaviours – and they lost weight.

- Not only did people lose weight, but they also became less depressed and anxious as a result of the increases in their behavioural flexibility.

- They also kept the weight off effortlessly, and felt happier and healthier. Their relationships improved too.

- Work by other researchers has shown that creating new behaviours to replace old ones can dramatically reduce the risk of developing cancer and heart disease.

CHAPTER FIVE

Stop Dieting, Start Living

Bad habits are like chains that are too light to feel until they are too heavy to carry.

Warren Buffet, billionaire investor and business guru

Welcome to your new life! This probably sounds a bit glib, but it's not meant to be. This chapter really is the start of your new life, one where you are finally in control of your weight. If you've started this book at the beginning and read it through methodically, you'll know that your habits shape and control you. We are all driven by our habits – both good and bad. As the ancient Greek philosopher Aristotle said, 'We are what we repeatedly do.'

How to follow the programme

The *No Diet Diet* programme is split into five parts or 'phases'. The first four should take you about one week each. Don't worry if they take a day or two longer, the important thing is that you complete the tasks in the order they're given. Please remember that it's better to do each phase well over nine days rather than badly over seven. You should, however, do your best to complete each one of them in

> • As well as helping you lose weight, the *No Diet Diet* is good for you because: *the weight loss is permanent.*

the allotted seven days. This will maximise the weight loss. The final phase is designed to embed all of the progress you'll have made during the previous four weeks. And it's just as interesting and inspiring as the first four phases.

If you're going to achieve your aims, you will have to commit yourself to following the *No Diet Diet*. That's all we ask. If you follow it completely, then you're virtually guaranteed to lose weight.

The *No Diet Diet* may look simple (it's certainly simple to do), but it has been carefully honed through many years of painstaking research. With this in mind, please carry out all of the steps

The power of friendship

Never underestimate the power of friendship. You may find it even easier to do the *No Diet Diet* with a friend or colleague. This can help you overcome two barriers to successful habit-breaking in one leap. Mutual support is a reassuring way of *Doing Something Different*. But not only that, it will help you overcome any concerns your friends may have about the *No Diet Diet*.

Many of your habits and behaviours will be partly kept in place by other people. They probably expect you to behave in the same old ways because that's what you've always done. But don't let that stop you from trying new things. Just get the other people on your side. Talk to them about what you're doing and why you're doing it. Tell them this is the best chance you have of getting what you want. And that, in the long run, it will benefit everyone because you'll be happier and healthier. You never know, they might even want to try it as well.

So why not encourage your friends and family to follow the *No Diet Diet* too? You'll get far more out of the programme if you do it with others. And while you're at it, why not set up a *No Diet Diet* club of your very own?

carefully. Some may look frivolous, but they all have a far deeper meaning than is immediately apparent, and will pay handsome dividends over the coming days and weeks. Here's a brief overview of the five phases of the *No Diet Diet*.

Phase One: Preparation

Phase One lays the groundwork for habit-breaking. Every time you break a habit, you weaken your habitweb and take a crucial step along the road to weight loss. To do this, all we ask you to do is:

- **Carry out one simple task each day, such as spending 15 minutes writing down your thoughts and feelings, or giving up watching television for a day.**

- **Perform two extra tasks over the course of the first week. You can choose which days to do these. They aren't too oner- ous and involve such things as listening to a different radio station or going to the cinema by yourself.**

Phase Two: Daily habit-breaking

Have you ever noticed how infectious a smile is? If someone smiles at you, it's almost impossible not to smile back. The way we behave towards each other is gov- erned by many deep-seated habits. These are so strong and ingrained that they mas- sively limit our free will. In fact, some psy- chologists claim that behavioural habits

• As well as helping you lose weight, the *No Diet Diet* is good for you because:
it's scientifically tested and founded on sound psychological principles.

are so powerful that we have virtually no free will at all – we just think we do.

If you spend a few minutes watching yourself in your mind's eye, you'll notice that a lot of your behaviour is a reaction to what other people are doing. Often this behaviour is not inherently *bad*, but it shows just how much you're constrained by your habits. Smiling may be a good behavioural habit, but you probably have many others that are bad – or at least restrict your room for manoeuvre. You'll find that, in any given situation, you will naturally react in only a limited number of ways. This reduces your adaptability and curbs how much you get out of life. It means that you're always reacting to what other people are doing rather than charting your own course through life. In order to pick your own path through life, you need to break your behavioural habits so that you can *choose* how to act rather than being constantly railroaded off in one particular direction by your habits. And this is where Phase Two kicks off. It helps you break the habits that govern how you *behave* in day-to-day life. Once again, *Doing Something Different* ensures that you get something different. You'll no longer be a rat on a treadmill destined to endlessly repeat your past mistakes.

> • As well as helping you lose weight, the *No Diet Diet* is good for you because:
> *it replaces your bad habits with good ones.*

To achieve this, all we ask you to do is behave a little differently each day in seven key personality areas (or behavioural dimensions):

- **Assertive–Unassertive**
- **Calm/Relaxed–Energetic/Driven**
- **Definite–Flexible**
- **Spontaneous–Systematic**
- **Introverted–Extroverted**

- **Conventional–Unconventional**
- **Individual-centred–Group-centred**

The aim is to break your habits in these areas. Don't worry, we'll explain more about these terms and their significance later on.

How you'll do it

Over the course of a week, we'll give you seven new things to do – one for each day. Again, these are simple and straightforward. For example, if you are normally an unassertive or laid-back person, we ask you to be a little more assertive in putting your views across. This is not to get you to expend energy in a heated argument. It's simply to break the habit of always behaving in the same way. That's it! During Phase Two you can expect to lose around another 2 lb (1 kg) in weight.

Phase Three: Changing habits and seizing back control of your life

Phase Three is where you'll subconsciously start to become far more mentally flexible and less habit-bound. If you suffer from food cravings, they will begin to subside. You will no longer be attracted to unhealthy food. You'll become filled with energy and, once again, begin experiencing the best that life has to offer. You can also expect to lose a further 2 lb (1 kg) in weight.

Phase Three involves looking in more detail at your habits and measuring their negative effects on your life. You'll do this by working your way through a few brief questionnaires. These short 'life quizzes' allow you to fine-tune the No Diet Diet to suit yourself. It's far simpler to do than it sounds and is incredibly effective. The emphasis is still on losing weight by making life more interesting. In short:

- **You'll need to carry out one simple task each day. These are designed to break the habits surrounding how you interact with people. You'll see how small changes ripple through your colleagues and circle of friends.**

- **You'll also need to carry out two additional tasks through-out the course of the week. You'll pick these from a menu of new activities. These include such innocuous tasks as throw-ing something away that you no longer need, turning off your mobile for a day, or going for a 30-minute walk.**

Phase Four: Targeting problem areas to continue your transformation

This is the stage where your most ingrained negative habits final-ly begin blinking out of existence one by one. As your old habits melt away, you subconsciously adopt a new and healthier way of living. Again, this is completely natural and effortless but, more importantly, it's fun! At the end of Phase Four you are likely to have lost around 7–9 lb (3–4 kg) since you started the *No Diet Diet* (and whatever your weight loss, your life will be improving in many other ways too).

Phase Four targets your subconscious thought patterns. For most people, how they think and behave is governed by how they thought and behaved in the past. Yes, even our thoughts can be driven by habit. When this happens, you can all too easily become trapped by the past and, in the process, lose control of your weight.

Phase Four tackles mental habits, which frequently trap us in negative ways of thinking. Do you always, for example, feel depressed and guilty when a diet fails you? The thoughts that cause depression, anxiety and guilt are all too often governed by habit. Phase Four helps you break the habits buried deep inside your subconscious. You will not be aware of these habits – so deep are they buried – but they govern much of what you think and feel. These habits must be broken if you are to get the best from the *No Diet Diet*. Phases One, Two and Three begin the process. Phase Four completes it and allows you to change your deepest thought processes so that they work *for* you rather than *against* you.

> • As well as helping you lose weight, the *No Diet Diet* is good for you because: *it deals with the* whole *person*.

Once this process is complete, you'll be infinitely more flexible and adaptable. You will no longer be driven by your old habits. You will no longer be trapped by your past. You will be absolutely free to make the best decisions possible. In practice, you will no longer be caged inside a vicious cycle of dieting (and getting nowhere). Instead, you'll lose weight effortlessly and be all set to maintain your new body for life.

To kick-start this deeper transformation, each day we'll ask you to:

- **Act in a different way towards somebody.**

- **Behave differently in a normal daily situation.**

We'll guide you through this process so that it's easy and fits neatly into your daily life.

Phase Five: Embedding your progress for life

One of the most surprising things about the *No Diet Diet* is that weight loss continues long after the initial 28-day programme has been completed. This is because virtually all of our clients' most damaging habits have been broken. If you complete the first four phases of our programme then you will continue steadily losing weight for many weeks and months afterwards. But this weight loss may eventually stall as a new set of bad habits gradually takes over your life. Phase Five prevents this from happening. It's not a rigid step-by-step, or day-by-day programme. It's a collection of tools that allows you to embed habit-breaking into your daily life.

> • As well as helping you lose weight, the *No Diet Diet* is good for you because: *it isn't based on restriction or self-denial.*

These tools include a monthly habit-spotter questionnaire. The idea is for you to sit down with a friend and spot each other's habits before they gain undue influence over your life. There are several other tools too. These encourage you to *Do Something Different* as often as you can. And as you know, the secret of staying slim is to continue breaking your habits by *Doing Something Different.*

And finally …

Before you leap headlong into the *No Diet Diet* we have a few questions for you. This will help clarify your thoughts and allow you to get the most from the programme. It should take less than two minutes. Consider each question carefully and circle 'True' or 'False'. It's usually best to give the first reaction that comes into your head.

1. I like to stick to the things I know best.
    True / False
2. I don't like to try new things.
    True / False
3. I don't see any good reasons to change the way I am.
    True / False

4. I have faults, but there is nothing I really need to change.

   True / False

5. I am not the kind of person who changes much.

   True / False

6. I don't think I need to develop myself and try new things.

   True / False

How did you do?

If you answered 'True' to only one or two questions (or none at all) then you are ready to embark on Phase One of the *No Diet Diet*. This means you are ready and able to take on and successfully complete the programme.

If you answered 'True' to three or more of these questions then you'll need to open yourself up a little more to habit-breaking. Please do not think you have failed. You have not. You have discovered something very important about yourself, which will allow you to precisely tailor the *No Diet Diet* to your own needs. You don't *fail* any part of the programme, you simply do not maximise your progress. Every step you take – even if you think you've *failed* it – eases the transition into a new, slimmer you.

If you did answer 'True' to three or more questions then you will need to do a little more work on making yourself open to change. And the simplest way of doing this is to start Phase One of the *No Diet Diet*. Once you've completed this, re-do the questionnaire. You are virtually guaranteed to have made the required progress. If this is the case, then you are ready to start Phase Two. Many people think that they cannot change and are afraid of trying new things. Phase One shows that you can break habits and open yourself up to fresh ways of thinking, feeling and behaving. As we've already explained, it is this process that encourages weight loss.

So, to recap:

- If you answered 'True' to either none, one or two questions, then start Phase One of the *No Diet Diet*.

- If you answered 'True' to three or more questions, then start Phase One of the programme. When you've completed it you should re-do the questionnaire on page 62 to check up on your progress and see how you've changed.

KEY POINTS

- The *No Diet Diet* programme is split into five parts or 'phases'.

- The first four phases are designed to break the habits that govern and control how you *do* things, how you *behave* and the way that you *think*. Break these habits and you will naturally shed 7–9 lb (3–4 kg) in weight over the course of the 28-day programme.

- You can expect to continue losing weight for many weeks and months after completing the programme.

- Phase Five embeds habit-breaking into your daily life. It ensures that you'll continue shedding your excess weight until your body's natural healthy weight emerges. It also ensures that your bad habits never again control your life.

CHAPTER SIX

Phase One: Preparation

Nothing is stronger than habit.

Ovid

OK, we won't beat about the bush. Here's what you have to do to get the weight-loss ball rolling:

- There is a separate page for each step of the *No Diet Diet*. **This will tell you what to do on that day.**

- **Try and do the tasks you are set. It's important that you don't miss out *any* steps. You should aim to do one step each day so that Phase One is carried out over one week. There is a space at the top of the page for you to fill in the date so you can help keep track of your progress.**

- **If you do have to skip a day – and can't manage to do the steps consecutively – don't worry. Just carry on where you left off as soon as you can. However, breaking the programme will lessen your chances of success. And remember, you do need to do all of the steps.**

- **There are also two additional tasks to complete before the end of Phase One. If you're in a rush, please don't be tempted to do the tasks half-heartedly. There's no point cheating yourself.**

Lucy, 28, lost 11 lb (5 kg) on the *No Diet Diet* and is now her ideal weight. Despite her success, she almost fell at the first hurdle. Giving up TV for a night was the greatest challenge she faced during the whole of the *No Diet Diet* programme.

'I thought giving up TV would be impossible. I spent the first hour wondering how I could spend my time. It felt weird. I got over it by looking in the mirror and imagining how I'd look if I was 10 lb (4.5 kg) lighter. That gave me the determination to keep the TV switched off! I knew that if I could do that I could do anything.

'Then I phoned my mum and spent an hour chatting to her. I found that once I was moving I quickly forgot about the TV. I cleaned the house, sorted out the airing cupboard, threw away my diet books and even started planning a holiday. I finished off the night by pampering myself with a long, slow bath. I filled the bathroom with candles and sprinkled some "sugar and nectarine" bath oil on to the steaming water. I had a wonderful relaxing night and achieved far more than if I'd just watched the TV. The only hard part about switching off the TV was making the decision. After that it was easy.'

Step 1   Date

Your task for today is:

Don't watch the TV – all day! If you're not a TV viewer, cut out the radio

This may be difficult, but please make sure you do it. Slumping in front of the TV is a habit that you've probably acquired without think-ing. We are *not* saying that watching TV makes you fat.* But we are saying that being trapped by your habits means it's infinitely harder to lose weight. And watching TV is a particularly potent habit. You know the feeling well: you come home from work, sit down, turn on the TV and watch it. And watch it. And watch it. You know there are other things to do, but somehow you just can't bring yourself to do them. So you watch TV. And tomorrow night you'll watch the TV again. And the next night. And before you know it, you're a couple of stones heavier.

Apart from a few good programmes, an awful lot of television is actually quite boring. The problem is, we've all got so used to watch-ing it without thinking. Consciously watching the TV is one thing, slumping comatose in front of it is quite another. Research shows that watching the telly is a mindless activity that allows your habits to maintain their stranglehold. Real pleasure comes from active engage-ment with life. Believe it or not, the majority of people say they get more satisfaction from work than they do from watching television!

* Although, in 2004, Professor Manfred Spitzer, a neuroscientist at the University of Ulm in Germany, found a direct correlation between watching excessive amounts of television and death caused by obesity, high blood pressure, high cholesterol levels and diabetes.

Watching TV can suck away your life without you noticing; when you switch it on, you switch off. Unless you're actively enjoying a programme – and engaging with it – the hours you spend in front of the TV is dead time. You've lost that time and it will never return. Please ask yourself this question: Is television really so jam-packed with gripping programmes that you can't switch it off for a day?

Instead of collapsing in front of the television, why not spend a few moments thinking about the other things you could do instead? You'll quickly notice that you have an awful lot of extra time you can use for other things. So, why not do one of your weekly tasks? And while you're at it, why not use some of your extra time to phone a friend or relative? Isn't time spent improving a relationship so much more positive than mindless viewing?

And the best thing is, you'll have just used the time to break a habit and lose a little weight!

Your other tasks this week: *Do Something Different!*

Over the course of the next week you should do two activities from the list below. Choose two that you wouldn't normally do or feel comfortable carrying out. The idea is to do *new* things so that you break habits and get out of your comfort zone. It's easy to do some of the tasks without any effort. But the more effort you put in, and the more different it is from your norm, the more you'll benefit from the *No Diet Diet*.

Now, tick the two things in the list that you want to do. And remember, don't choose the things that you normally do!

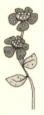

NEW THINGS TO TRY	WHEN WILL YOU DO THEM?	TICK WHEN DONE
1. **Newspaper:** change it or stop buying one.		
2. **Magazine:** buy and read a different one.		
3. **Radio:** change channels or start listening to it again.		
4. **Food:** try something you've never eaten before. Be adventurous!		
5. **Journey:** go somewhere new or take a different route to a familiar destination, such as work or your favourite seaside town.		
6. **Public meeting:** go to the local town hall or somewhere else where there's a meeting.		
7. **Sport:** It can be anything. Why not try yoga, table tennis, cricket or swimming?		
8. **Paint or draw:** use pens, pencils, paints or charcoal – whatever you wish.		
9. **Watch a live sports event:** choose any event and go and watch it.		
10. **Charity work:** choose any local group and go and help out.		
11. **Domestic chores:** do something new. It doesn't matter whether it's the washing-up or some DIY.		
12. **Read:** choose something you wouldn't normally consider. It doesn't matter whether it's an obscure book or a trashy magazine.		

NEW THINGS TO TRY	WHEN WILL YOU DO THEM?	TICK WHEN DONE
13. Write a story: any subject, any length.		
14. Exercise: do something different.		
15. Cinema: go by yourself to watch a film.		
16. Contact a long-lost friend or relation.		
17. Shop: go somewhere different.		
18. Museum or exhibition: visit any one.		
19. Shift: sit in a different place to your usual one. This could be at mealtimes, in the lounge, at meetings, anywhere where you have your 'habitual' place to sit.		
20. Improve your spelling: use a dictionary to learn ten new words.		
21. Broken friends: make the first move to repair the damage.		
22. Ride a bike.		
23. Play a child's game. Hopscotch anyone?		
24. Learn to meditate.		
25. Drive in a less aggressive manner (a tough one for some!).		

Step 2   Date

Your task for today is:

Write something for 15 minutes

Make sure this is something you wouldn't normally write (no shopping lists allowed). A story perhaps, or a poem, or maybe the start of your own life story. Would today be a good day to start keeping a diary? Writing is a great way of focusing your mind. Over time it helps clarify the way you want to live. You might feel that you don't have a book inside you, but there will certainly be many ideas that you'd like to get down on paper. Why not describe the person you want to be in a year's time?

The most important thing is to begin. We know from bitter experience that the most difficult part of writing is actually scribbling down the first words. So just start, even if it seems like you are writing random words, it doesn't matter. Look out of the window, what do you see? What does your room look like? Why not start a story by weaving together the last three conversations you had. Don't worry, nobody need ever see what you've written. Bury it at the bottom of your sock drawer, if you wish.

By writing for 15 minutes you've taken another step towards breaking your habits, freeing your soul and losing weight!

Common excuses used for *not changing* – or why people say they can't *Do Something Different*!

- I don't adapt to change very easily.
- There are too many things going on in my life at the moment for me to change.
- I'll change when my circumstances improve.
- If I had more time (or money, or friends, or room) I could change.
- My past stops me from changing in the way I'd like to. My childhood (because of social or money worries) stops me from changing.
- Other people stop me from changing. I need to look after my children (or partner or parents), so I just don't have the time or the energy.

How many of these do you recognise in yourself? These are thinking habits that can all too easily get in the way of your aims. Once you recognise them for what they are – just habits of thinking rather than real reasons – you can begin to move on. Change isn't only possible, you've already started! In just 25 days' time you can be a different, slimmer person just by continuing with the *No Diet Diet*.

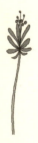

Step **3**   **Date**

Your task for today is:

Don't have your favourite drink

If you drink tea, coffee or fizzy drinks, don't let a drop pass your lips today. Why not try an alternative? Avoid the coffee machine and head for the water cooler instead.

Does your body react to not having its favourite drink? Caffeine withdrawal is quite common. This is partly a sign of chemical addiction, but it also signifies your body's rebellion against the breaking of a particularly powerful habit.

The tea and coffee habit is particularly hard to break. For many years now, you've probably been endlessly repeating the same tea and coffee habits. Like most people, you probably fall out of bed in the morning, stumble into the kitchen, and put the kettle on. Breaking this habit sends a little shock through your system. There will be many times today when you unconsciously reach for the kettle. Breaking this habit will deal a particularly powerful blow against the habitweb.

Many people end up like laboratory rats, forced by their habits to endlessly repeat the same actions over and over again. Rats are often driven by their habits to run around their exercise wheels for hours on end (which is at least healthy). Many people, on the other hand, have probably spent years reaching for the kettle, the TV remote control and the diet book. It doesn't matter whether these habits are

> • As well as helping you lose weight, the *No Diet Diet* is good for you because:
> *it doesn't disconnect you from your appetite or destroy your natural ability to recognise whether or not you are hungry.*

pointless or damaging. The habitweb is driving you and the only way out is to break your habits one by one.

Your other tasks this week

OK, we don't want to nag you, but … have you done either of the two additional tasks yet? You need to tackle them soon because there's only a few days left. If you have, well done! Make sure you tick the list.

Step **4**   **Date**

Your task for today is:

Go for a 15-minute walk. Think about your life and what you want from it

It's important that you make time for this walk and don't just incorporate it into your normal routine. You may have to plan it a day or two in advance so that you are able to fit it in.

If you're a morning person, it might be worthwhile getting up a little earlier to go for the walk. If you're not, then all the more reason to break out of your comfort zone and be an early riser, even if it's just for one day. Or you could try fitting it into your lunch hour. We've found that for many people the best time is straight after work. If this is the case, plonk all of your stuff down when you get back home and head straight out again. This should prevent you from immediately settling back into your habitweb.

Walking is a fantastic stress reliever. We were all born to walk! Don't feel you have to rush anywhere. Take your time. This is 15 minutes of pure thinking space. After a few minutes, you'll probably notice how it clears your head. Do you still feel tired and muggy? Do you feel re-energised?

One of our clients, Joshua, became an avid walker after starting the *No Diet Diet*. For over 20 years he'd been a dedicated couch potato. But the act of walking completely reinvigorated Joshua's life. He started off reluctantly walking for 15 minutes as we advised. The next day he decided to do it again. He now just potters around his local neighbourhood every night after work. It's his private thinking space.

What happened next didn't just surprise Joshua, but us too. Apart from losing 2½ stone (16 kg) in weight, it reconnected him with his seven-year-old son, Peter, who suffers from Asperger's Syndrome, a form of autism. After a while, Joshua began taking Peter on his daily walks. Although Peter suffered from learning difficulties, and had some behavioural problems, he soon started looking forward to his daily walks with his dad. Very quickly his behaviour improved markedly. Over the course of a few months, Peter turned into a new boy. And his behaviour is continuing to improve. It was an unexpected benefit of the *No Diet Diet*.

Joshua told us, 'The *No Diet Diet* has affected every part of my life. Every day, I try to do something different. It is simple and quite profound. I tell everyone I know about its benefits. Yes, I've lost weight, 2½ stone (16 kg) so far, but to me what's most important is that I've started to live again.'

Joshua's story shows that although some of the tasks we've asked you to do can seem trivial, they can have extraordinary consequences. Small changes can start a cascade of events that takes you to a far more positive place. Weight loss is just one of the many benefits of the programme. But first you have to continue taking small steps away from habit-world.

Please read me!

Tomorrow's task is to get up an hour earlier than normal, so don't forget to set your alarm clock tonight! After your little walk, you might feel like going to bed an hour earlier too.

Your other tasks this week

Have you done either of the two additional tasks yet? You need to do so soon. If you've done them, tick the list.

Step 5

Date
_____

Your task for today is:

Get up one hour earlier

Bad habits find the mornings cosy, warm and extremely accommodating. Many people find it inordinately difficult to get going in the morning, so it's all too easy to rely on habits to keep you moving. This is a very fertile time for your most ingrained bad habits. Analyse your own behaviour. If you're like most people, you'll stumble out of your bed, put the kettle on, brush your teeth and get washed with your eyes half closed. Like a robot, it's all too easy to perform a set of pre-programmed routines. Your morning routines have become rigid because you don't have a spare minute to consciously think about what you're doing.

If you set the alarm for as late as you can get away with, you'll start the day all hurried and hassled. You'll have barely enough time to accomplish what you need to do. You'll be on the back foot from the second you open your eyes. This means you'll always be reacting to events rather than seizing the initiative. So get up earlier and take control of your life!

When you get up early you have a headstart over all of your tasks, troubles and worries. If you have more time, it's easier to change your routines and break your bad habits. So today you should change your usual morning habits. You should spend more time on the things you'd normally rush through. You could use the hour to eat a leisurely breakfast. Try sitting down and enjoying it rather than eating it on the hoof. Why not have some freshly ground coffee instead of instant, a cup of leaf tea instead of a bag, a nice long bath instead of a quick dash under the shower? Why not walk to the newsagent's

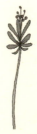

and buy a morning newspaper? On the way, spend a little time noticing how much goes on while you're normally asleep. Watch the simple beauty of a sunrise. See how the light slowly spreads across the world. Watch the frost melt or the dew evaporate. Observe how the morning slowly changes from deep shadow to bright crispness (or perhaps dank greyness). Early mornings can be quite stunningly beautiful.

• As well as helping you lose weight, the *No Diet Diet* is good for you because: *it expands your life rather than restricts it.*

There are lots of ways you could use this extra hour. You could do something around the house, prepare for the day ahead or catch up on some reading or letter writing. Try and break your normal habits and shake up your usual routine. If you usually have breakfast before getting dressed, then why not put your clothes on first today? If you usually leave the dishes in the sink for later, why not clean them up? If you normally have the TV on as you're getting ready, why not put the radio or a CD on instead? Just make sure you try and do something different.

The aim of today is not to deprive you of your sleep. Instead, we're trying to show you that you can make changes in your life, even if at this stage they're only small, subtle ones. Remember, this is just the start of the *No Diet Diet*. These incremental transformations are laying the groundwork for permanent changes – and permanent weight loss.

All of the activities in the *No Diet Diet* are designed to make you wake up to the habitweb. They will make you aware of the things you do every day without thinking. Almost anything you can do can be driven by habits. By becoming aware of your habits – and breaking them – you create the right conditions for permanent change to occur.

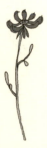

Although today you've only made a few new decisions, you might feel slight twinges of unease creeping in. This is your habitweb trying to draw you back into its fold. Always doing the same things over and over again is comforting. But it's also a trap. Breaking the habitweb's grip in small ways weakens it. Every day that passes – every new deci-sion you make – weakens your habitweb and strengthens your will.

You should now congratulate yourself. Today you've taken a big step forward!

A gentle prod

Have you done either of the two additional tasks yet? If so, tick the list. If not, choose the two now and decide when you will do them this week.

Step 6

Date

Your task for today is:

Make a list of what you want to achieve by this time next year

The bigger your dream, the more your life will change. But write down the small things too.

Focusing on your goals means that they're more likely to happen. Here are a few questions to help you concentrate your mind, but please remember, they're your dreams and ideas, so feel free to write down whatever you want. Here goes:

- **How much would you like to weigh next year?**
- **How would you like your personal relationships to develop over the coming year?**
- **Where would you like to live?**
- **How do you see your career developing?**

Now make a list of the concrete steps you can take to achieve these goals. It needn't be long. Don't worry if they seem daunting – you don't have to put them into action immediately. The idea is to get you thinking freely and to banish all of your excuses. If you wish, you can add to this list in the future. You can also add to your list of dreams whenever you want to. Start to dream and never, ever stop! And if you can banish the habit of making excuses, you'll make huge progress.

Your other tasks this week

Have you done the two additional things yet? You need to do so by the end of tomorrow. If you have, tick the list.

Step 7   Date

Your task for today is:

Do a good-natured deed for someone else, one that could change their life a little for the better

A random act of kindness is the most magical gift you can give to anyone. So, your task for today is to do a small good-natured deed for someone else. It needn't be something big. Perhaps you could help a workmate tidy their desk, help a neighbour carry their shopping or do something that you know your partner hates doing. If you've finished a good book, why not leave it on a park bench or bus seat?

Think about your friends, family and workmates. How can you make their lives a little bit better? We guarantee that there is one small thing that you can do for someone else that will improve their whole day. It might involve giving just for the sake of giving, without expecting to receive anything in return. Perhaps if you know a colleague is hard pressed on a particular job you could leave a little treat on their desk first thing in the morning. If an elderly person near you lives alone, why not give them your phone number in case of emergency? Try not to tell anyone else about it. You'll be paid back in other ways.

Many years ago, I sprained my ankle in the street. A teenager came out of the barber's shop where he worked and helped me to a chair. He then gave me a cup of coffee. For him it was such a simple thing, but it brightened up my whole day. Now the only thing I remember is the gratitude. The pain is long forgotten. If you see someone needing help today, why not give them a hand? If you don't see someone in need, why not simply leave a bunch of flowers on a workmate's desk?

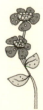

We don't want to nag, but ...

Have you completed your additional tasks? You need to do so by the end of today. Make sure you tick the list!

Phase One assessment: how did you do?

Q. How many of the seven steps did you do?

    1   2   3   4   5   6   7

Circle how many you did. Multiply this number by three and write your score here:

. . . .

Q. How many of the two additional tasks did you do?

               1   2

Circle the number you did, double it and write your score here:

. . . .

Add the two scores together and write your total here:

. . . .

Q. Did you take a break in the week? (i.e. did the seven steps take more than one week to complete?)

If *yes*, deduct four points from your total.

Write your new total here:

. . . .

How did you do?

Scored less than 15

You are not yet ready to proceed with the rest of the programme. In order to achieve your goal, you'll need to make changes in your life. Our score suggests that you haven't managed to do this yet. Remember: *you have not failed*! Nobody *fails* the *No Diet Diet*. You have simply not maximised your gains. Why not have another go at Phase One and see if you can improve your score? This time you could try doing it with a friend, family member or online at www.HabitDoctors.com or www.nodietdietway.com. And remember, if you follow the *No Diet Diet* you will lose weight!

Scored 15 to 20

Well done! You've made a good start. However, before you can move on to Phase Two you need to do one more task today. This can either be one of the seven steps that you might have skipped, or you could try one of the additional tasks. Do this now and you'll be well on the way to your goal. You should then move on to Phase Two.

Scored 21 or more

Congratulations! You've done very well in your first week and shown that you can make significant changes to your life. You have a great chance of reaching your weight-loss goal. Try to keep up your resolve as you go into Phase Two.

KEY POINTS

● Phase One lays the groundwork for long-term habit-breaking. Every time you broke a habit, you weakened your habitweb and took a crucial step along the road to weight loss.

● You should have completed the seven steps in one week. If you didn't manage to do this you may have reduced your overall weight loss. However, don't feel you have failed – you have not. But please try and complete Phase Two in seven days. If you do this you will maximise your rate of weight loss.

● Most people lose around 1 lb (0.5 kg) in weight during Phase One, but many people lose more.

CHAPTER SEVEN

Phase Two: Weight Off for Good Behaviour

Man becomes a slave to his constantly repeated acts. What he at first chooses, at last compels.

Orison Swett Marden

Our research shows that, on average, people lose around 1 lb (0.5 kg) in weight during Phase One. But that's not really the primary aim of this phase. It's about laying the foundations for *healthy sustained weight loss so that you never have to diet again*. And this is what will happen over the coming weeks. Phase Two is where you'll start moving forward in leaps and bounds. It's the point where you'll start making concrete changes that will embed weight loss into your life. Phase One created the conditions for change. Phase Two puts it into practice.

Now to weight loss – which, after all, is the reason why you're doing the *No Diet Diet*. There are plenty of diets that claim you can lose 6–8 lb (3–4 kg) a week, though, in reality, you'd be lucky to lose 2–3 lb (1–2 kg). But these diets lead to intense food cravings, anxiety, guilt and depression. You can never sustain such a diet for long, because neither you nor anyone else has the willpower to put up with the mental and physical punishment it entails. As a

> 'Studies show [the *No Diet Diet*] works just as well as Atkins and Weight Watchers – if not better – when it comes to helping you lose weight. And you don't have to read a single food label.'

result, the weight loss is temporary and pretty soon after abandoning the diet, you'll weigh more than you did before you started it. This leads to guilt, depression and yo-yo dieting.

Every time people go on a diet they're convinced that this time they'll succeed. This feeling is so common that psychologists even have a name for it. It's called 'false hope syndrome', and it's experienced by people who diet time and time again, even though they always fail. They're always convinced that *this time it'll be different*. It never is, of course. The only way to get something different is to *Do Something Different*.

With the *No Diet Diet* you *are* capable of losing 1–2 lb (0.5–1 kg) a week until your ideal healthy weight emerges – and of keeping it off for life. What's more, the *No Diet Diet* will deliver this weight loss without hunger pangs, depression or guilt, so we hope you'll agree that it's worth persisting with it through Phase Two and beyond.

> • As well as helping you lose weight, the *No Diet Diet* is good for you because:
> *it doesn't focus on food so you don't become obsessed by it or develop an unhealthy attitude towards it.*

Katy, one of our earliest clients, gave up halfway through Phase Two on her first attempt. A few weeks later, she tried again and found that everything clicked for her on the second attempt. She found that, as time went by, it became increasingly easy to make changes in her life. She's now more than 2 stone (15.5 kg) slimmer, which is about where she wants to be. Her advice? 'Keep doing something different. Just remember where you want to be in a year's time!'

The bonus for Katy is that she knows she'll never have to go on a food diet ever again.

Good behaviour

By now you've probably accepted the fact that habits govern a large part of your life. Phase One showed you that you had a number of physical habits which determine the way you actually go about *doing* things. Watching the television, drinking tea and coffee, brushing your teeth are all, to a large degree, governed by *doing* habits. You do things a certain way because you've always done them that way.

Now for something a little more shocking. What if we told you that your habits also controlled how you behave and interact with other people? Doesn't that send a shiver of despair down your spine? Well, we've got some interesting news for you – habits really do control how you behave. That's one of the major reasons why you're overweight. You probably have very little control over how you behave day to day. *But you can have!* The essence of the *No Diet Diet* is to hand you back full control over your life. And it'll happen sooner than you think.

But first, we'd like to prove to you how much of your present life is manipulated by the habitweb. Just spend a few minutes running through a typical day in your mind. We'll wager you a pound to a penny that a huge number of the things that you do in a typical day are simply repeats of what you did yesterday, the day before, the week before that, the month before ...

Here are a few examples: Do you always sleep on the same side of the bed? Get up at the same time? Do you always have sex on the same nights of the week (and in the same positions)? Do you always go to the toilet at the same times? Do you always take the same number of footsteps to the bus stop, station or car? Do you always take the same route to work? And, when you're there, do you always drink out of the same mug? Do you always sit in the same chair at meetings? Do you always have the same polite conversations with the same people? Need we ask any more?

You can see how much of your behaviour in a typical day is

controlled by habit. One habit leads inexorably to the next, which triggers the next, and the next. Of course, we're all fully conscious and aware of what's going on around us. It's just that we tend to do the same things over and over again. It feels comforting somehow. It's a personalised Groundhog Day.

Many habits are innocuous, of course. They help us automate certain parts of our life. Nobody, for example, wants to overly contemplate switching on the light when they just want to banish the dark. But other habits, particularly those relating to food and exercise, can be very harmful. As can relationship habits – always falling for the same type of loser – always feeling that *you* are the only one who can change them. Research has shown that our behaviour towards food, relationships – in fact, just about everything – is governed by habit.

So is it any wonder that, when you try and change one habit by going on a diet, all of the others claw you way back into their web? You're not just fighting the urge to eat. You are fighting *everything*! Brute force will not spring you from this prison. To escape, you'll need a little bit of cunning. You'll need to break your habits by stealth. You'll need to *Do Something Different*. And this week we'll do this by asking you to *behave* slightly differently to the way you do normally.

Over the next week you will be given seven tasks that will enable you to explore the different parts of your character. In doing so, you'll break some of the most powerful and ingrained habits of all. The parts of your personality to be explored are:

• As well as helping you lose weight, the *No Diet Diet* is good for you because: *it's a means of grabbing hold of your future, not being a prisoner of the past.*

- **Assertive–Unassertive**

- **Calm/Relaxed–Energetic/Driven**

- **Definite–Flexible**

- **Spontaneous–Systematic**

- **Introverted–Extroverted**

- **Conventional–Unconventional**

- **Individual-centred–Group-centred**

You will see that each personality area has an opposite, and that together they form the opposite ends of a behaviour spectrum. Most people tend to operate within a very narrow part of this spectrum. For example, if your partner is grumpy one morning, there are many ways for you to react. Responding with exceptional warmth and compassion is at one end of the spectrum. Outright hostility lies at the other. In between these two extremes are a million possibilities. Most people – largely because of habit (which also drives temperament) – will react in only one way. Some of the time this will be the best way. But most of the time it will be the behavioural equivalent of using a sledgehammer to crack a nut. As the old saying goes, 'If the only tool you have is a hammer, you will see every problem as a nail.' The aim of Phase Two is to break your behavioural habits by adding some more tools to your toolbox. Hammers are not the only tools!

In Phase Two we'll ask you to behave slightly differently to the way you do normally. You should view this as a licence to explore different parts of your personality, the parts that have become a little rusty through underuse. See it as acting. You get to cast off your old clothes and try on some new ones. It doesn't have to be forever, you can try it out just the once. At first you might like to try it out in a small and subtle way so that no one notices. When you do this, you'll see that you get a subtly different response from other people. They probably won't even be aware of how they've changed in response to you. You will have become a catalyst for change, not just for yourself, but to those around you too. Perhaps you've always wished a certain person would behave differently? See what happens when *you* act differently towards them. Remember that if you *Do Something Different* you get something different in return.

Some of the things we'll ask you to do in Phase Two may at first seem a little vague. This is because you'll be asked to reflect on parts of your own character, which can take a little thought (but don't worry, it's not too difficult). For example, in Step 8 we'll ask you to evaluate the degree to which you are assertive or unassertive. Some people find this confusing because they are not sure where they fit on the spectrum. How they view themselves may also differ from how their friends and family see them. If this happens to you, then you should trust your own judgement. Even if you are a little unsure about it, just go with your first gut feeling. The important thing is to make a decision and act on it. There really is no absolute right or wrong answer. It genuinely makes no difference whether you score four rather than five on the assertiveness spectrum. The aim is simply to find roughly where you normally fall on the spectrum and then to behave differently.

If you score zero on the spectrum, or are completely unable to decide, then here's a little trick to help you arrive at an answer: Look carefully inside yourself and see what makes you feel least comfortable. Does the prospect of acting more assertively for a day make you feel slightly uneasy inside? If this is the case then you should assume that you are 'naturally' unassertive so you should aim to be more assertive for the day.

At the end of Phase Two you'll have lost around 2 lb (1 kg) and be far more flexible and adaptable. Your habits will have far less control over you, and you'll be far less stressed and hassled by daily life. You'll be in the driving seat – not following the wishes of everyone else around you. You'll be cool when it pays to be cool, passionate when you want to be, and relaxed the rest of the time.

One important point to remember, though. When you try behaving a little differently you must make sure that it's appropriate to the situation. It may be advisable to scream and shout at a mugger, less so in a business meeting.

When you begin Phase Two, you may feel like you've changed gear. This is because you'll have to start choosing different ways of behaving from a list of options, rather than relying on us to tell you what to do. This is how we precisely tailor the *No Diet Diet* to your needs. It's another way that it differs from food diets and one of the main reasons it works. This isn't as hard as it at first appears and you'll only have to make one small change each day.

Step 8

Date

Your task for today is:

Be more (or less) assertive

Today you get to work on assertiveness and unassertiveness. These are obviously two very different ways of reacting to a situation. Both are legitimate in their place, but you may have fallen into the habit of *always* being too assertive or unassertive (or of never being either). If the world really is a stage, today you get to play a different role.

But first, what do we mean by assertiveness and unassertiveness?

- **Assertive** is insisting upon your rights, or asking for what you want.

- **Unassertive** is not putting yourself forward, not asking for what you want.

  How do you rate yourself? (And remember it's how you feel about yourself that counts, not what other people think.) Place a tick on the scale below ...

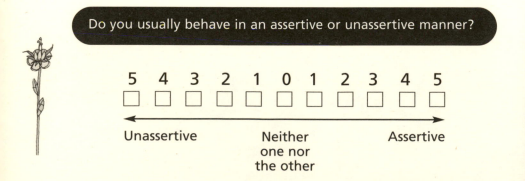

Do you usually behave in an assertive or unassertive manner?

5	4	3	2	1	0	1	2	3	4	5
☐	☐	☐	☐	☐	☐	☐	☐	☐	☐	☐

Unassertive　　　　　Neither　　　　Assertive
　　　　　　　　　　one nor
　　　　　　　　　　the other

As you have probably guessed by now, consistently being too much one way or the other is not a good idea.

Being consistently *too assertive* can make you appear aggressive and unwilling to take into account other people's views. This can harm your career, as people may dislike working or doing business with you. It may also harm your social life, as people may feel you're too pushy.

Being consistently *too unassertive* may result in you never getting what you want. It may also mean that you consistently let others make decisions for you. This can damage your career, as your bosses may feel that you don't look after the company's interests sufficiently well. Socially, some people may feel that you are too shy and retiring to be good fun to hang around with. In a relationship, your partner may think you're something of a pushover, as may your children.

There are obviously varying degrees of assertiveness and unassertiveness in between these two extremes, and a myriad of acceptable alternative ways for you to behave. Cast your mind back to the assertiveness scale you ticked a few moments ago. Today you should try behaving more in the opposite manner. Today you should *Do Something Different*.

Putting it into practice

During the course of today, situations will crop up where you would normally react assertively or unassertively. Try to anticipate some of these. Think about when they might happen and how you would normally respond.

If you are normally assertive

Do you always have something to say about what's being discussed? Are you one of those people who has an opinion on everything? Today, even if it's just for a short period of time, try sitting back and being unassertive. Then, just observe what happens. Pick one of these options (tick one) or come up with one of your own ideas:

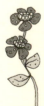

❏   **Stay in the background more.** For example, if you're in a meeting don't blurt out your feelings. Try watching how the situation develops and do your best not to influence the outcome.

❏   **Ignore criticism, *don't react* to it.** For example, if you're on the phone to a lecturing relative or friend, why not bite your tongue. Remember this is the perfect opportunity to put the *No Diet Diet* into practice.

❏   **In a discussion or meeting, behave as if another person knows better than you (even if they don't).** If you can't bring yourself to agree verbally, why not nod and smile? You're not committing yourself. This is just an exercise.

❏   **Let somebody else choose or decide for you.** This can be a relatively small decision, such as allowing somebody else to choose your sandwich. You never know, you might like it.

❏   **Or think of your own way of being unassertive and write it here:**

If you are normally unassertive

Today you could try being more confident and direct with someone. Pick one of these options (tick one) or come up with one of your own ideas:

❏   **Be direct in asking for what you want.** This could be at work or socially (even in bed). For example, you could tell your friends which pub or restaurant you'd like to meet in.

❏   **Express an opinion.** This could relate to politics, a work issue or the state of the global environment. You choose.

❏ **Be more forceful in putting across your views on an issue you believe in.** If during conversations you normally express an opinion sheepishly and leave it at that, today why not argue? Why not counter the other person's viewpoint with one of your own. You don't need to be aggressive but you do have the right to your opinion, whether it's at home, in the office or out with friends.

❏ **Say no (when it's OK to).** For example, if you're out with friends and everyone wants another drink, but you don't, then say no. Likewise, if everyone wants to leave the pub you're in, but you don't, why not ask them to stay a little longer?

❏ **Or think of your own way of being assertive and write it here:**

Step 9

Date

Your task for today is:

Change how you behave in a group

To a greater or lesser extent we're all social chameleons. The character we adopt in a group can differ from how we are when we are alone. A great example is during family gatherings. At Christmas, birthdays, weddings and funerals, virtually everyone slips back into the role they've played most of their lives; it's extremely difficult not to revert to the character everyone expects you to be. You know the feeling: if you're the youngest, nobody can quite accept that you're no longer five years old. And, to a degree, you play up to their expectations. The same is probably true for almost every group you belong to. Whether it's at work or out socialising, your 'group' persona is likely to be highly habit-bound. It's vital that you break these habits and today that's what you're going to do.

When you're in a group, do you normally focus primarily on yourself, or do you put the others first? Both are acceptable ways to live your life, but it's all too easy to fall into one pattern of behaviour. That's not only bad for you, but it also means that you are a less effective member of the group, so, ironically, you can all lose out in the end.

But first, what do we mean when we talk about being group-centred or individual-centred?

- **Group-centred** means taking a team view or going along with the group. It's putting the needs of the group first, whether they are family, friends, team members or the organisation you work for.

- **Individual-centred** means doing your own thing and putting yourself or your own needs before those of the group.

  As you can probably guess, it's not good to behave consistently in the same way.

- **Being too individual-centred may make you appear inconsiderate or selfish, with the result that people neither trust nor like you. This could harm your career prospects and limit your social life.**

- **Being too group-centred may mean that you don't do what's best for you, or for the other groups to which you belong. It may also mean that people take advantage of your good nature. Paradoxically, it may harm your career because you don't get noticed as an individual or recognised for your good work, with the result that you're constantly overlooked for promotion.**

  It's possible – and legitimate – to adapt your behaviour as circumstances dictate. In fact, interacting with a group provides a great opportunity for you to break habits and behave differently. When in a group, people often focus on themselves. This means that you can change your behaviour without it being too obvious. And this change could trigger a different reaction from others without them even realising it. Try it and see for yourself.

How do you rate yourself? (And remember, it's how *you* feel about yourself that counts not what other people think.) Place a tick on the scale below ...

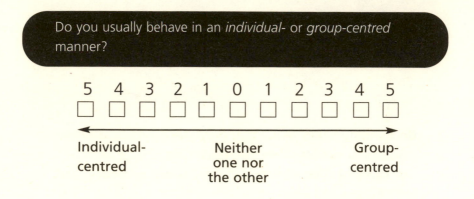

Do you usually behave in an *individual-* or *group-centred* manner?

| 5 | 4 | 3 | 2 | 1 | 0 | 1 | 2 | 3 | 4 | 5 |
| □ | □ | □ | □ | □ | □ | □ | □ | □ | □ | □ |

Individual-
centred

Neither
one nor
the other

Group-
centred

Putting it into practice

During the course of today, situations will arise when you would normally focus mostly on your own interests or those of the group. Try to anticipate some of these and behave in a different way.

If you are normally a group-centred person, try to be more individual-centred

Please remember, though, the idea is not to be selfish (a horrible trait, we feel), but to consider your interests as much as you consider those of the group. Sometimes putting yourself first can benefit the group. For example, if you're a busy mum or dad who always puts the family first, you may resent not having enough time for yourself. Resentment is corrosive. Giving yourself a little time to be yourself may do wonders for the wellbeing of the family as a whole. It will ensure that you are happier and more content. This will make you a far better (and more effective) mother or father.

People are often group-centred because it's the easy option. So today, even if it's just for a short time, pick one of the options given below (tick one) or come up with one of your own ideas:

- **Take an individual stance.** At work, for example, don't put any more effort into a task than your colleagues are doing. If it's a group task, everyone should pull their weight. You shouldn't over-work yourself so that others can get a free ride.

- **Share your individual needs with one or more members of the group.** For example, if you're out for dinner with friends and need to leave early you should tell everyone early on. Don't feel you need to apologise. Simply state your needs. You'll be surprised by the response.

- **Do the right thing without asking others.** If you know the answer to something, then make a decision without getting the OK from other people. Don't feel that you need to apologise to them for taking a stand that accords with what you know to be right. Just do it.

- **Do something purely for yourself.** It's important that you take time every day to be kind to yourself. If you're rushed doing group work, for example organising a social gathering, take some time for yourself to do whatever you want. If you want to go shopping, or to the pub with your mates, just do it. Don't feel guilty. You've earned it.

- **Or think of your own way of being less group-centred and write it here:**

If you are an individual-centred person, try being more group-focused

Remember, the aim is to try and put the interests of the group before those of yourself. Don't worry, you won't need to make huge sacri-fices and you'll quickly find that helping others often indirectly benefits you. You'll find that if you make the first altruistic move, peo-ple will often fall over themselves to help you in the future. Helping

others also induces a warm feeling of satisfaction that helps reduce stress and boosts the immune system. Pick one of the options given below (tick one) or come up with one of your own ideas:

❏   **Offer support or help to another group member.** If someone is clearly falling behind with their work, why not offer to do some of it for them? They'll be eternally grateful!

❏   **Organise an event that all of the group can take part in.** For example, your friends might like to go for a night out together. Why not organise it?

❏   **Listening and learning is fundamental to being part of a group.** So why not listen carefully to the suggestions of others? You never know, you might learn something.

❏   **Or think of your own way of being less individual-centred and write it here:**

_____

Step 10   Date

Your task for today is:

Change your energy level

Chilled out or hyper? People vary hugely in the degree to which they are calm or energetic. This not only varies according to personality, but also in relation to mood, time of day or the situation in which they find themselves. Even the calmest person may find it difficult to relax while stuck in a traffic jam for three hours. Likewise, even the most hyper-driven workaholic may find it difficult to get excited at the end of a particularly boring day at the office. Some people, however, can always be too relaxed in the way they approach things while others seem to be permanently hyper.

But what, exactly, do we mean by calm and relaxed or energetic and driven?

- **Calm/Relaxed** means being peaceful, not stressed and without tension.

- **Energetic/Driven** means being enthusiastic, motivated and bubbling with energy.

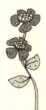

How do you rate yourself? (And remember it's how you feel about yourself that counts not what other people think.) Place a tick on the scale below …

Do you behave in a calm/relaxed or energetic/driven manner?

5 4 3 2 1 0 1 2 3 4 5
☐ ☐ ☐ ☐ ☐ ☐ ☐ ☐ ☐ ☐ ☐

Calm/   Neither   Energetic/
Relaxed   one nor   Driven
               the other

Putting it into practice
Today try to take a different perspective!

If you are normally energetic
Adopt a more relaxed approach to life. For example, pick one of the options given below (tick one) or come up with one of your own ideas:

☐ **Take five minutes out every hour to think about anything you choose.** And we mean anything! It could be your next holiday, a potential partner, a beautiful work of art, or your dream house or car. Of course, if you insist, you can think about work.

☐ **Do something *slowly* instead of rushing through it.**

☐ **Put something off until later.** This could be the washing up, paying a bill, returning a phone call, or updating the office spreadsheet. It really doesn't matter what you do so long as you use the opportunity to slow down.

☐ **Think about why you're tackling the task that you're doing.** Ask yourself if it's important. If it isn't, why are you doing it?

❏   **Let yourself be bored – don't fight it.**

❏   **Or think of your own way of being less energetic and write it here:**

_____

If you are normally a relaxed person

Try to be more driven. For example, pick one of the options given below or come up with one of your own ideas:

❏   **Take on a new role or activity.** This could be at work (become a fire warden or a first-aider, for example) or it could mean taking on a new hobby.

❏   **Take 20 per cent less time over everything you do.** Try to shop, work and walk a little faster. Keep asking yourself: 'Can I do this quicker'. Write these words on a note and stick it on your desk, TV, purse or wallet. Or why not post a copy of it to yourself?

❏   **Do something you've been putting off for a long while.** This could be paying a bill, visiting a sick relative, or taking a day trip to a castle or the seaside.

❏   **Take the initiative when you'd normally leave it to somebody else.**

❏   **Or think of your own way of being more driven and write it here:**

_____

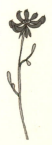

Step 11   Date

Your task for today is:

Optimise your flexibility

Is flexibility a good thing? Generally speaking, yes. Being flexible ensures that you can spot opportunities as they arise, which in turn means you can make the most of life. It's also true that flexible people are generally slimmer than those who are less flexible – that's why increasing behavioural flexibility lies at the heart of the *Do Something Different* philosophy. However, being *too* flexible can also be a bad habit. There are times when being overly flexible can prevent you from getting what you want. Having definite ideas about what you want out of life – or what you're trying to achieve – makes them infinitely more likely to happen. So when it comes to flexibility, the best way to behave is to have definite ideas about where you want to go with your life, but to remain flexible in how you achieve your goals.

In practice, this means that if you have a tendency to consistently behave either flexibly or inflexibly then you'll miss out on many opportunities, including the chance to lose weight. Behaving consistently one way means you'll only ever get one result (or variations of it). Adapting to suit the circumstances means you'll achieve what you want, whether that's losing weight, getting a new partner or winning a promotion.

What do we mean by being flexible or definite?

- **Definite** means being certain, sure and decisive.

- **Flexible** means being open to change, willing and able to adapt.

   How do you rate yourself? (And remember it's how you feel about yourself that counts, not what other people think.) Place a tick on the scale below ...

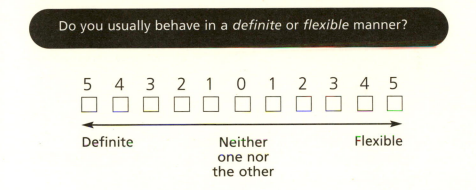

Do you usually behave in a *definite* or *flexible* manner?

5   4   3   2   1   0   1   2   3   4   5

Definite   Neither   Flexible
                           one nor
                           the other

Putting it into practice

Today you are going to be different!

If you are normally flexible

Try being more definite. For example, pick one of the options given below (tick one) or come up with one of your own ideas:

❏ **Adopt a stance and see the benefits of taking a firm line.** This may take the form of defending your point of view in work or in a relationship.

❏ **Don't be so accommodating of other people's views or actions.** Speak out if necessary. (It's best to do this only when you think it's appropriate, though!)

❏ **Make a strategic decision and act on it, instead of being swayed by the immediate circumstances you're in.** If you're out shopping for new clothes, for example, give yourself a budget – and stick to it come what may.

❑ **Pay more attention to the big issues, and don't allow yourself to be distracted by the smaller ones.** For example, at work it's very easy to be swayed by pointless bureaucracy and to lose sight of your actual job. Answering minor emails and phone calls can easily consume your entire working day, and more. Just remember that when you're dead your in-tray will still be full!

❑ **Or think of your own way of being more definite and write it here:**

If you are normally very definite

Try being more flexible. For example, pick one of the options given below (tick one) or come up with one of your own ideas:

❑ **Ask someone else how they see the issue you're dealing with.** Why not go further? Why not listen to their viewpoint and arguments, think them through, and then impartially see which is the best course of action? Then put this decision into practice.

❑ **Imagine you're on the receiving end of what you're about to do.** Then ask yourself, 'How do I appear to them?' You could try this at the supermarket checkout or on the phone to a call centre. You could also try it in response to an issue raised by your partner. The important point is to mentally step outside of yourself and observe how you behave.

❑ **On the hour, *every hour*, stop!** The idea is to catch yourself before you blindly carry on with what you're doing. Then ask yourself, 'Could I be doing something that's even better – something that takes me closer to my goal?' You should then ask, 'Am I doing this task in the most effective way possible?'

❏ **Let others be 'right' today, be humble, don't criticise.** We're not saying that you should blithely follow a reckless course of action. But you should allow others to carry out their wishes wherever possible. If they're wrong, well, it's not your fault. If they're right, then you'll have learnt something new. Sometimes not arguing and allowing others to make decisions can be very therapeutic. You should try this both at work and in your social life.

❏ **Or think of your own way of being more flexible and write it here:**

_____

> Remember: It's how you feel about yourself that counts. If you feel like a flexible person then you probably are. If this is the case then it's important to change your behaviour to become more definite. Listen to your friends and family but ultimately *you have to decide*.

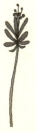

Step 12

Date

Your task for today is:

Optimise your spontaneity

Do you do things on the spur of the moment or do you systemati-cally work through every small detail before making a decision? As with all facets of the human character, people differ hugely in how spontaneous or systematic they are. That's what makes everyone unique and interesting.

There's nothing wrong with being either spontaneous or system-atic. Without both ways of thinking, society would quickly fall apart and civilisation probably wouldn't have got going in the first place. The problem – as ever – occurs when you consistently behave one way or the other. The trick to a happy and productive life is to be both as spontaneous and systematic as the situation demands.

OK, first, what do we mean by being spontaneous or systematic?

- **Spontaneous** means doing things on the spur of the moment.

- **Systematic** means planning and considering everything in advance in an orderly way.

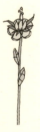

How do you rate yourself? (And remember it's how you feel about yourself that counts not what other people think.) Place a tick on the scale below ...

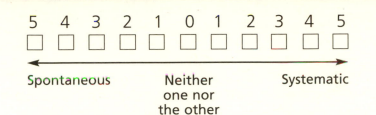

Do you usually behave in a *spontaneous* or *systematic* manner?

| 5 | 4 | 3 | 2 | 1 | 0 | 1 | 2 | 3 | 4 | 5 |

Spontaneous   Neither
                     one nor
                     the other   Systematic

Putting it into practice
Today try out a different approach!

If you are normally spontaneous
Try adopting a more systematic approach to one or two situations that arise today. For example, pick one of the options given below (tick one) or think of one of your own ideas:

❑ **Make plans now for something that's going to happen in the future.** It doesn't need to be in the far future. Tomorrow or next week is fine. Draw up a list of everything you need to do to make it happen. Then arrange those tasks in a logical order. Think carefully about every step that's required. Only when you've done this should you actually begin putting the plans into action.

❑ **Organise an area of your life that's too haphazard, anything from sorting out your CDs to putting your finances in order.**

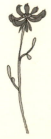

❑ **Make a list of the things you want to achieve over the next week, the next year and over the course of your life.** Make some notes on how you'll start to achieve these goals. File them away – yes, that's right, a file for organising things!

❑ **Timetable your whole day in half-hour slots.** Start by listing absolutely everything you plan to do that day. Then estimate how much time everything will take. The final step is to put the items in a logical order so that you can do them all in as efficient a way as possible. It'll actually make the whole day run more smoothly and you'll have loads more time on your hands.

❏ **Or think of your own way of being more systematic and write it here:**

_____

If you are normally systematic

Try being more spontaneous. For example, pick one of the options given below (tick one) or think of one of your own ideas:

❏ **Do something on the spur of the moment.** Flick through a 'what's on' guide and choose something that takes your fancy. You could try listing six things you'd like to do, give each one a number then roll a die to see which one you'll do. Or why not stick a pin in a map of your local area and visit it?

❏ **Ignore your plans and just do what feels right.** Close your eyes and see what you'd like to do. Go and do it without thinking. Just walk out of the door immediately!

❏ **Try something silly or frivolous – have fun!** Why not run down the street singing in the rain? Or why not visit a funfair, tell a stranger that you like what they're wearing or take up an adventure sport? These aren't commands – you should choose.

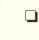

❏ **Tell at least two people how much you like them (and the *No Diet Diet*!).**

❏ **Let the day unfold without organising it, just see what happens.**

❏ **Or think of your own way of being more spontaneous and write it here:**

_____

Step 13   Date

Your task for today is:

Fine-tune your temperament

Are you a shy, retiring butterfly or boisterous like Tigger? How naturally outgoing you are was probably shaped, in part, by your childhood. As a result, it is likely to be incredibly habit-bound. The good news is, the more a part of your character is hedged in by habits, the more habits there are to break. And the more habits you break, the faster you'll lose weight. See it as a target-rich environment – as snipers say.

But before we show you how it's done, we just want to make sure that we're all singing from the same hymn sheet. What exactly do we mean when we talk about being introverted and extroverted?

- **Introverted** is being shy, inward-looking and not outgoing.

- **Extroverted** is being outgoing, boisterous and sociable.

Obviously, by now, you'll have guessed that it's not good to behave consistently one way or t'other. We can hear you asking, 'But how the hell do you change something as fundamental as being an introvert?' It's easy! The trick is to view yourself as an actor. Surprising as it may seem, many famous actors are incredibly shy and introverted. They overcome their shyness by giving themselves a licence – or permission – to behave differently. They step outside of themselves by adopting a role that's been crafted by someone else. Try it for yourself and see how effective it is.

So today you should give yourself a licence to behave differently.

The aim is to act in the opposite way to how you would normally. It can be fun and you'll soon appreciate the benefits of breaking this habit. When you break this one, which you will have done by the end of today, you will have taken a massive step forward.

How do you rate yourself? (And remember it's how you feel about yourself that counts not what other people think.) Place a tick on the scale below ...

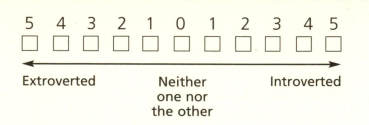

Do you usually behave in an *extroverted* or *introverted* manner?

5 4 3 2 1 0 1 2 3 4 5
☐ ☐ ☐ ☐ ☐ ☐ ☐ ☐ ☐ ☐ ☐

Extroverted   Neither   Introverted
                  one nor
                  the other

Putting it into practice
Today try being a different person!

If you think you are an introvert
Try being a bit more extroverted. For example, pick one of the following (tick one) or come up with one of your own ideas:

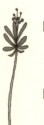

☐ **Contribute to a discussion when you wouldn't normally express an opinion.** If expressing an opinion is too big a step for you, then you could simply say when you agree with someone else.

☐ **Make the first move over a friendship.** For example, phone a friend just for a chat or invite someone for a coffee. Such simple moves can kick-start a budding friendship or relationship.

❑ **Get out of your shell.** For example, try talking to somebody completely new or someone you meet at an event. You could practise opening lines for when you meet new people. A good way of starting a conversation is to ask a question, this breaks the ice a little. Another trick is to ask people about themselves. This is especially true if you're afraid of not being 'interesting' enough.

❑ **Smile a little more.** A smile is always a great ice-breaker and it only uses half as many muscles as a frown. It instantly signals that you're an outgoing, kind and approachable person. And it automatically makes you and others feel good. And it's free! You could couple this with more open body language. For example, uncross your arms and use more expansive gestures. Try and make sure that you don't have clenched fists or look at the floor when you speak. You'll probably find that people then engage you in conversation. Before you know it, you'll be chatting away.

❑ **Learn one really good joke and when the right moment comes along, tell it.**

❑ **Or think of your own way of being more extrovert and write it here:**

_____

If you think you are an extrovert
Try being a bit more introverted. For example, pick one of the following (tick one) or come up with one of your own ideas:

❑ **Listen more and speak less.** Extroverts tend to dominate conversations. So, if you keep quiet for a while you'll instantly allow people to open up to you. Every time you feel the need to speak, hold your tongue for a few breaths while you carefully consider what you're about to say. You can speak but you shouldn't try and seize control of the conversation. You should also try and keep the volume down.

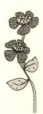

❏   **Spend some time alone.** Enjoy your own company when you would normally meet or phone a friend for a chat. This could be a sobering experience for you. It will give you a great opportunity to catch up with all of the other things you've been meaning to do over the past days and weeks.

❏   **Say no to a social invitation.** Stay at home or go for a walk. Just for one day, keep out of the limelight. You may find that it's quite a pleasant experience to spend some time with yourself.

❏   **Fade into the background a bit more.** Bite your tongue and don't comment on anything until you've carefully considered what you're going to say. Why not try being less flamboyantly dressed as well? The idea is to blend with the wallpaper for just one day.

❏   **Don't interrupt other people or finish their sentences.** A tough one for true extroverts.

❏   **Or think of your own way of being more introverted and write it here:**

_____

Remember: It's how you feel about yourself that counts. If you feel like an introvert then you probably are. If this is the case, then today it's important for you to change your behaviour to become more extroverted. Listen to your friends and family but ultimately *you have to decide.*

Step 14

14

Date

Your task for today is:

Try being more (or less) conventional

Being conventional and generally 'fitting in' is comfortable. It means that you don't have to think so much about your clothes, hair or make-up. Your views and tastes are catered for by big 'mass-market' companies and brands. In effect, all of society revolves around your needs and desires. This makes life easier, but it also serves as a trap … a fat trap!

In this area of our characters, context is everything. Some people move in circles where pierced tongues and tattooed faces are normal, whereas a balding middle-aged civil servant would appear distinctly unconventional at a Botox party. With this in mind, your next task becomes infinitely easier. Today you get to switch roles when it comes to being conventional or unconventional. But first, what do we mean when we use these terms?

- **Conventional** means being traditional, formal, behaving according to normal custom and generally 'fitting in'.

- **Unconventional** means being different, willing to stand out from the crowd.

How do you rate yourself? (And remember it's how *you* feel
about yourself that counts not what other people think.)
Place a tick on the scale below ...

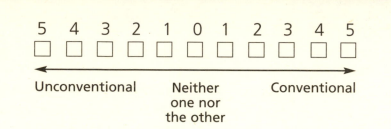

Do you usually behave in an *unconventional* or *conventional* manner?

5	4	3	2	1	0	1	2	3	4	5
☐	☐	☐	☐	☐	☐	☐	☐	☐	☐	☐

◄──────────────────────────────────►

Unconventional   Neither   Conventional
                       one nor
                       the other

Putting it into practice

During the course of today, situations will crop up where you would
normally react in either a conventional or unconventional way. Try to
anticipate some of these. Think about when they might happen and
how you would normally respond. Then try (if it's appropriate) doing
the opposite.

If you are an unconventional person

If you naturally resist going with the crowd, why not switch roles
today? After all, they're just flip sides of the same coin but arise from
equally rigid mind-sets. So, even if it's just for a short time, why not
try one of the following (tick one) or come up with one of your own
ideas:

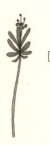

☐   **Make the more conventional choice instead of striving to be
different.** You may find it difficult to know what conventional is, so
just try to do what makes you feel the most uneasy. If your spirit
rebels, you're probably doing the right thing! For example, you
could try wearing different (and more conventional) clothes or

listening to more mainstream music. And while you're at it, why not do your hair in a more 'normal' way?

❏ **Consider the more traditional alternative and attempt to just fit in.** Try doing exactly what everyone else around you is doing. Imagine you're watching a natural history programme, study their behaviour and just copy them.

❏ **Conform by taking the easily acceptable option.** Whatever it is, be it politics, an office squabble or a family feud. Just go with the flow.

❏ **Agree with someone, even if you don't share their view.** Most people do this because it's easy, for you it's probably the most difficult thing in the world – but do it anyway.

❏ **Or think of your own way of being more conventional and write it here:**

_____

If you are generally a conventional person

Try being more unconventional. For example, pick one of the following (tick one) or come up with one of your own ideas:

❏ **Look at situations from a completely different angle.** How would a Martian view your position? The first step is to begin reacting as you would do normally, then stop, and do the opposite instead (but only if it's appropriate).

❏ **Wear something less conformist and mainstream.** Go shopping in a different place and try on all of the clothes you'd normally leave on the racks. Even if you don't buy them, when you look in the mirror and see a different you, it will make you realise how stuck in one image you've become. And who knows, it might give you some ideas to pep up your style.

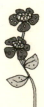

❏ **Take something in your life that's very ordinary and change it.** For example, you could focus on clothes, food or how you spend your leisure time. Why not choose food at random? Why not get a 'what's-on' guide for your area and study the sections you'd normally skip through. Why not wear odd socks – who said they have to match anyway?

❏ **Try to make more unconventional choices.** Every time you have to make a decision, why not ask yourself what feels 'nice and comfortable', then change it. It doesn't matter what it is. The idea for today is to be different. Go to the hairdresser's. Instead of having the usual, allow the stylist to do what they think will suit you. Remember, a change is as good as a rest.

❏ **Or think of your own way of being more unconventional and write it here:**

Step 14

NoDietVonni (we'd love to know who you are too!) kept an online diary of her experiences with the *No Diet Diet*. Not only did she lose two pounds during Phase Two but also increased her bust size by an inch, lost 1¾ inches around her waist, and an inch on her hips. Whilst she enjoyed doing the programme, she also found some tasks very challenging indeed. Here's what she wrote for Step 14:

'Today's task was to be more conventional. This is something I have a difficulty with, considering I am:

- of ethnic minority;
- fairly heavily pierced;
- overweight (hey, if I wasn't, then why the hell would I be doing this?!?!)

I geared myself up to taking out all my visible piercings, bar a sleeper in each earlobe. That meant taking out six in my right ear (three lobe, three pinna), one from my right ear (one lobe), and my lip ring.

As soon as I removed the piercings, I was stricken with anxiety. I did not want to go outside and have the world see me like this, this plain, mousey-looking frump. Walking to the top of the road was horrible – I felt ugly and exposed. I thought people could see through me and see I wasn't the person I make out to be, but I knew I couldn't go back.

I seriously thought it would not make a blind bit of difference as to how people treated me. But I was wrong. It did make a difference. I felt ignored. Invisible. People just treated me as if I didn't exist. As if I didn't matter. Like anything could happen to me and it wouldn't matter because I was a non-person. That scared me more than being gawped at like I'm from Mars.'

So how do you feel?

We hope you've enjoyed the past two weeks. We also hope that there's slightly less of you. Around 2–4 lb (1–2 kg) less, in fact. Our research has found that once people embark on the *No Diet Diet* they tend to lose 1 per cent of their body weight *every week*. So if you weigh 150 lb (6.8 kg) then you can expect to lose around 1½ lb (680 g) every week. And this is maintained until your ideal healthy weight emerges. This is the ideal rate of weight loss recommended by doctors around the world.

Take a little peek ten weeks into the future. You'll be carrying significantly less fat around with you. You'll also be feeling slimmer and happier. Given that the *No Diet Diet* achieves this weight loss without food cravings, anxiety or guilt, we think that our programme is the ideal way to lose weight. Please forget about crash diets, they simply inflict immense damage on your body and guarantee that you'll yo-yo back to where you started from. The *No Diet Diet* is the healthy way to lose weight. And this weight loss is maintained until your ideal healthy weight emerges.

You may also have noticed several other unexpected benefits. Your relationships may have improved. Anxiety and depression will be reduced. You've probably started to think about de-cluttering your life and focusing on what is important to you. While these are all important, you may also have noticed that your diet is improving of its own accord. This is because, deep down in your soul, you know what's good for you. As soon as your unhealthy habits begin to break,

> 'I lost 2 lb (1 kg) at the end of the first week and I also received lots of other unexpected benefits from the programme. I never watch the TV, so I had to give up the radio for a day. I normally listen to it when I drive to work. Instead, I took the time to plan my day whilst waiting in traffic jams. I found that it makes me arrive much less stressed and far more prepared for the day ahead.'
>
> Jemma, 32

inner strength and knowledge emerge from the wreckage. And it's these that will guide you over the coming weeks.

Bad old days

Compare these gains to how you'd feel on a conventional diet. At the end of the second week, you'd probably feel tired, depressed and washed out. You would have wasted huge amounts of time counting calories, or avoiding carbs, and agonising over which was the best, GI or GL. As a consequence, you'd be wracked with insecurity, food cravings and guilt. Virtually every waking moment would have been filled with thoughts of food. Every day would have been a battle of wills. And one you were destined to lose.

If you were lucky, you'd have lost 6 lb (2.75 kg) in weight on a conventional food diet by now. But that would be largely an illusion. Most of the weight loss would be water. As the days passed, the rate of weight loss would start to decline. 3–4 lb (1.5–1.75 kg) in the first week would decline to 2–3 lb (1–1.5 kg) in the second. After a month – if you lasted that long – weight loss would decline to around 1–2 lb (0.5–1 kg) a week. And the worst part would be to come. As the lack of energy began chewing into your soul, you'd begin to fail. The first sign might be an extra biscuit sneaking into your diet, or perhaps sugar slipping back into your tea or coffee. If you were being particularly 'lax' you might have used full-fat salad dressing rather than the reduced-calorie variety. This 'failure' will have made you feel guilty. Once again, you will have entered a vicious cycle of failure. And each time you failed, your willpower will

'The rate of weight loss given sounds slow but is actually quite sensible and it's more likely to stay off than some quick-fix solution followed in the short term.'

Sue Baic, of the British Dietetic Association

have weakened a little bit more, making the next transgression infinitely more likely.

But the psychological impact would be only part of the problem. As your body struggled to make do with fewer calories, it could also become starved of vital nutrients. This would make you insatiably hungry – only a saint could resist! You may also start to feel light-headed and sleepy. In the long run, lack of calories, protein, essential fats and vital nutrients may even start damaging your body's major organs. And deeper inside you, and in the longer term, the damage could even kill you. Repeated dieting reduces the level of cancer-destroying natural killer cells.

Aren't you glad you opted for the *No Diet Diet* rather than the latest 'wonder diet'?

KEY POINTS

● Habits govern not only how you go about doing things but also how you behave. Phase Two started the process of breaking these behavioural habits in seven key personality areas.

● You should have lost around 2 lb (1 kg) in weight during Phase Two. If you haven't, don't worry. For some people, breaking the habitweb takes a little longer.

● The *No Diet Diet* encourages healthy, sustained weight loss that is permanent. Weight loss of 1–2 lb (0.5–1 kg) per week is ideal. And if you change your habitweb for good, which you will, the changes are permanent.

● You will probably also have noticed several pleasing side effects of the *No Diet Diet*. You'll probably feel happier, less anxious and more contented with life.

● Compared to food diets, the *No Diet Diet* is healthy for both your mind and body. There are no negative cycles of failure. There's no 'false hope', only positive personal growth and sustainable weight loss. Beat that, Dr Atkins!

CHAPTER EIGHT

Phase Three: Changing Your Habits and Doing Things Differently

If you have always done it that way, it is probably wrong.

Charles Kettering, American inventor

Phase Three of the *No Diet Diet* is where you really start moving forward in leaps and bounds. Don't worry if you feel that the programme is suddenly going to get a lot harder, because it isn't. In any case, you've already proved that you can make the necessary changes allowing you to lose weight. Phase Three is where you begin building on these changes. Our research shows that it's in Phases Three and Four that most progress is made and the majority of weight is lost. And this weight loss is both healthy and sustained.

We hope that after two weeks or so on the *No Diet Diet* you feel energised and full of life. You'll probably feel relaxed and happy, and imbued with a sense that life is filled with opportunity and purpose. In our studies, virtually everyone who's made it this far feels at ease with life and is determined to make even more progress. They've also lost a pleasing amount of weight. But the best is yet to come.

Phase Three builds on the foundations of Phases One and Two. This week, you'll get to peek inside your mind a little more, to learn about how you think and behave in relation to other people and your daily life. You'll get to tailor the *No Diet Diet* just for yourself. We hope you won't feel this is too onerous. The worst we'll ask you to do is make a child laugh or listen more carefully to another person's conversation. But more of that later.

By now you will have noticed just how many habits you have. Many of them you probably weren't even aware you had. Your

'When I was a kid, my mum and dad didn't have a car, so we used to walk everywhere, but it's one of those things you just get out of the habit of doing. On one of my "Doing" days I forced myself to go for a walk. I haven't walked anywhere for 20 years, so I thought going for a 30-minute walk would really be doing something different!

'My walk surprised me. I did it after work and found it completely relaxed me. The first five minutes were hell. I really didn't want to do it. I was huffing and puffing like a pit pony. But when I reached the park I realised how beautiful it was. The lake was full of ducks. The spring flowers were just opening. The birds were singing to each other. I was surprised at how being close to nature calmed and relaxed me.

'By the time I reached home I felt quite good about myself. Now I go for a walk three or four times a week. I walk to the local shop instead of jumping in the car. Sometimes I walk the dog for my neighbour; he's an old man whose health isn't too good at the moment so he's glad of the help. Now whenever life gets the better of me I tramp the streets until I'm relaxed. I just wish I'd re-discovered walking years ago.

'My advice to other "non-dieters"? Pick something you would never normally consider, maybe something your parents forced you to do when you were a kid, and go for it! You may enjoy it but even if you don't at least you will have opened your mind and lost a little weight.'

Emma, 38

task in Phase Three is to identify some more. Each day you should slice away one of these habits by doing something different. The focus will remain on the habits that govern how you 'do' things and the way you 'behave'. Although you will have already broken many of these habits in Phases One and Two, we still need to work on these areas a little more.

DO SOMETHING DIFFERENT: BATHS

When you take a bath is it just another routine thing in your life? Have you got into the habit of trying to do everything quickly, including washing?

What do you usually put in your bath? If you, like most people, buy a large bottle of coloured liquid from the supermarket to squirt in, then why not do something different next time? Did you know it's possible to get bath bombs, bath salts, bubble bath, bath cubes, bath oil, bath candy, bath float, aromatherapy bath oils, large tea bags filled with scent and herbs, milk baths and stress-busting bath liquids?

Our friend and agent, Sheila Crowley, is an amazingly successful and busy lady, but still finds time for a bit of pampering. She told us about Float Away, a wonderful bath essence that creates the feeling that you're actually floating on water while flooding your senses with heady, fragrant scents.

Why not set aside an hour for your next bath, play some music, light a few candles and carefully choose what fragrance, fizz or foam you're going to add to it? While you're at it, why not scatter real flower petals on the surface? Or you could add ice cubes for some pleasant sensations on a warm summer's night. You'll experience a mind-blowing reawakening from simply breaking a rather mundane everyday habit.

Preparing for Phase Three

To prepare for Phase Three, you'll need to think about some of the habits you have in relation to the people around you and the way you live your life. To do this, we've prepared two short 'life quizzes' for you. These should take only a few minutes each to complete. The idea is to pinpoint the number of habits you have in specific areas. These quizzes give you a score, which is then used to tailor the *No Diet Diet* specifically for you. You just look up your score on a simple table. This tells you the number of days over the following week that you'll need to devote to either interacting with people or trying out new things. We'll go into a little more detail on this later on. You should aim to do all of your tasks over seven days. This will maximise the gains. If you don't manage this, then just pick up where you left off as soon as you can. But the longer you leave it, the slower your progress will be. Under no circumstances should you think you've failed. Remember, you don't fail the *No Diet Diet*! You just don't maximise your progress.

In addition to these daily tasks, you'll need to do two extra ones over the same seven days. You should choose these from a list of 26 we'll give you later. And that's it. If you are experienced at calorie or carb counting, Phase Three will be a doddle.

Preparing to *Do Something Different*

Now we'd like you to think about some of the habits you have in relation to People and Doing things in everyday life.

People habits

Tick the box each time you answer 'Yes' to a question.

1.   Do you tend to react to all people in the same way? ❑

2.   Do you rarely start a conversation? ❑

3.   Do you see the same people all of the time? ❑

4.   Do you avoid people that are not like you? ❑

5.   Do you judge people quickly? ❑

6.   At a party, do you wait for others to say things? ❑

7.   Do you hold grudges against people? ❑

8.   Are you quick to see other people's faults? ❑

9.   Do you find it hard to give compliments to other people or to praise them? ❑

10. Do you think that you could never be friends with people who are different to you, either socially or politically, or who hold different views to your own? ❑

11. Do you think it is unnecessary to be polite to other people? ❑

12. When things go wrong, is it usually because of other people? ❑

13. Do you think that other people should contact you when it's their turn? ❑

14. Are there other people with whom you just can't get along? ❑

15. Do you avoid taking up issues with other people? ❑

16. Do you think some people are just not worth talking to? ❑

17. Are some people just lucky to be where they are? ❑

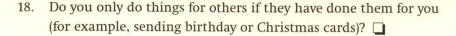

18.   Do you only do things for others if they have done them for you (for example, sending birthday or Christmas cards)? ❏

19.   Do you have people in your life whom you've fallen out with? ❏

20.   Do you ignore people who are not important to you? ❏

21.   Do you have only a few friends? ❏

22.   Do you keep confidences or secrets? ❏

23.   Do you feel jealous at the good fortune of your friends? ❏

24.   Do you relish the opportunity to gossip about people? ❏

25.   Are you ever rude to other people? ❏

DO SOMETHING DIFFERENT: TEA

Every little thing is habit-driven. Take something as simple as a cup of tea. A quick supermarket scan revealed that a typical local supermarket stocks over 180 different types and makes of tea. That's tea in bags, loose tea, energy-plus teabags, skin-purifying teabags and every flavour from camomile and spearmint to Lapsang Souchong. Did you know there are even ayurvedic de-stress teabags, after-dinner mint teabags and teabags for hard water?

Yet most people probably buy the same old standard teabags every week. They would say that's because they like those best. How do they know? Even in such a simple area of our lives, it's another example of how habit-bound we become. Why not change your tea habit and try something different?

How did you do?

Be totally honest here. How many of the above questions did you answer 'Yes' to? Make a note of your score (low, medium, high).

Scored less than 5   low

You don't appear to have too many bad People habits. This might be true, or you may be unaware of the habits that you do have. As you know, the first step to breaking habits is realising you've got them. So long as you've answered truthfully, you're doing well when it comes to People habits.

Scored between 5 and 10   *medium*

Like most people, you have a range of habits relating to how you view others and how you behave towards them. These, like other habits, are stopping you from getting what you want. You have to change them to lose weight. The more you can change these habits, the closer you'll be to achieving your goal.

Scored more than 10   high

You've recognised that you have too many thinking habits relating to the people around you. This is a sound basis from which to progress because you already know the areas in your life that need changing. Now, wherever possible, you should focus your attention on the habits highlighted by the questions you've just answered.

Doing habits

Now we have to work out how many habits you have in relation to Doing things. You'll be surprised by this one. But first, you'll need to work your way through this little quiz. Tick the box each time you answer 'Yes' to a question. After you've completed this, you'll almost have finished preparing for Phase Three.

1.   Do you often say that you are going to do something and not get around to doing it? ☐

2.   Do you tend to react to situations as you have done in the past? ☐

3.   When you have to make a choice, do you do nothing rather than make a decision? ☐

4.   Do you have a backlog of things you should have done? ☐

5.   Do you think that being different is something that other people can do but you can't? ☐

6.   Do you think that you don't have the time to do the things you'd like to? ☐

7.   Do you think it's too late to have the kind of life you'd like? ☐

8.   Do you worry about what other people will think if you start to do things differently or behave in a different way? ☐

9.   Do you think that it's not easy to fit into your daily routine the things you really want to do? ☐

10.   Do you ever say one thing and do another? ☐

11. Are you put off by the idea of doing what you think is right? ☐

12. Do you think it is impossible to get enjoyment from ordinary daily activities, such as gardening and housework? ☐

13. Are you bothered about the reactions of other people? ☐

14. Do you tend to do things the same way? ☐

15. Are you the kind of person who stays in the background and prefers not to be noticed? ☐

16. Do you smoke, or drink too much alcohol? ☐

17. Do you try to get others to do things for you? ☐

18. Do you think you were born the way you are and that it's difficult to do things differently? ☐

19. Do you think of yourself as having a strong personality? ☐

20. Do you have natural ways of doing things? ☐

21. Does the day often fly by? ☐

22. Do you think it's difficult to change? ☐

23. Do you often go on holiday to the same place? ☐

24. Do you have regular nights for doing things? ☐

25. Do you usually mix with the same people? ☐

How did you do?

How many of the above questions did you answer 'Yes' to? Make a note of your score (low, medium, high).

Scored less than 5   *low*

You don't appear to have too many bad thinking habits in relation to Doing things. This means it should not be too difficult to increase the variety of activities that you're happy to take on. This is great news! You could start off by addressing those questions that you answered 'yes' to, these could be the habits you need to try and break first.

Scored between 5 and 10   *medium*

You have a moderate number of thinking habits that limit your flexibility in how you 'do' things. It's important that these habits are broken. And this is what you'll do over the next week. You're on the right road to achieving your aims.

Scored more than 10   *high*

You recognise that you have many thinking habits relating to Doing things. This is a good basis from which to progress because you can already see the areas in which you need to improve. Onwards and upwards!

What do you do next?

Look up your scores (low/medium/high) for the People and Doing questions that you did a few minutes ago, then look at where they lie in the table shown below. This will tell you what you have to do during Phase Three.

For example, if you scored *high* on the People questions and *low* on the Doing questions, then you should do one Doing day and six People days during Phase Three. Or, if you scored *low* on the People questions and *low* on the Doing questions, then you should do three Doing days and four People days.

It doesn't matter which days you do them on, so long as you do the right number of each type of task over the next seven days. Again, if you miss a day, try and pick up where you left off as soon as you can. Breaking or not completing Phase Three will lessen your chances of success and slow down your weight loss.

Doing and People matrix			
	Low Doing Score	Medium Doing Score	High Doing Score
Low People Score	3 Doing & 4 People Days	5 Doing & 2 People Days	6 Doing & 1 People Days
Medium People Score	2 Doing & 5 People Days	3 Doing & 4 People Days	5 Doing & 2 People Days
High People Score	1 Doing & 6 People Days	2 Doing & 5 People Days	3 Doing & 4 People Days

People days

On these days you should try out different ways of interacting with people. The aim of these days is *not* to change your character or 'brainwash' you, it's simply to momentarily snap you out of the rut you've found yourself in. You'll find that if you behave slightly differently with the people you normally interact with, in a positive rather than a negative way, then these people will in turn become more interesting to you. You'll see a new and more intriguing side to their character. They will also look upon you in a new and more positive light. This will set off a virtuous circle that will significantly improve your life and relationships. Remember that the guiding principle of the *No Diet Diet* is to *Do Something Different*, so that you get something different in return. By breaking the habits surrounding how you interact with people, you'll be taking a step closer to achieving your aim, that is, losing weight. See your People days as 'change is as good as a rest' days.

Now, choose between one and six of the tasks given below depending on the table on page 137. Tick the ones you think you want to do (don't worry, you can change them later).

❑   **Listen** Take the time to listen to what people say, rather than guessing before they finish. You should try and concentrate 100 per cent on what they are saying. Don't butt in, interrupt or finish people's sentences. And don't try to offer solutions to their problems. You'll gain infinitely more by concentrating on what a person is actually saying, rather than focusing on what you want to say in response. Your reward will be a greater understanding and empathy for the other person's point of view. Why not go even further? Instead of saying something yourself when they've finished, ask them to tell you more, or to clarify or expand.

Ask Don't hold back in asking for what you want. If you want to know something, ask. Don't just pretend you already know. Never assume that you have all of the information you need. If you have the slightest doubt, seek clarification. And while you're at it, why not also ask your friends and colleagues some personal questions so you can understand them a little better? Ask a happy person how they stay so cheerful. Ask a colleague how they would spend their ideal weekend. Or just ring some-one up and say, 'I've always wanted to ask you this ...'

Give Give something away today. Give compliments, give of your time, but, most importantly, give without expecting to receive. If you give, you will receive. If you know what you want from other people, you are more likely to receive it if you offer it to them in the first place. For example, if you want respect, try giving it first. If you show appreciation for something, you are more likely to get a better job done next time. If you want more contact with friends, give them a call and make the first move. And if you want more affection, try giving it and see what comes back.

New Make a new friend, try something new with a friend, or try a new approach with a person you've never managed to get along with. If you carry on doing things in the same old way you will get more of the same in return. Don't be afraid of try-ing something new – the old ways are not necessarily the best. In fact, they are almost certainly the reason you need to make changes. Try a new approach, especially if the old one isn't working. If nagging at the kids is getting you nowhere, try smil-ing and ask politely for their help – your new demeanour could shock them into action.

Find Out Take the trouble to find out something new about a person you know, discover why your friends like you, or uncover a way of improving yourself. We all have blind spots, discovering

where they lie is the key to personal development and getting
what you want. Many people don't know what they are igno-
rant about. Why not attempt to discover some of your blind
spots today? Try and find out a little more about yourself, your
job, or your colleagues. This can only lead to new insights,
which will be immensely valuable. Or buy a book from a charity shop on an obscure but fascinating subject and learn more.

❏   **Help** Do something for someone, offer your assistance, or be
useful to another person or living creature. Helping others to
know and develop is beneficial to everyone. Do not try and keep
valuable knowledge to yourself. It will not give you the edge.
Sharing and helping produces the best outcome for all in the
long run. Look around you for people needing help. If one of
your friends has been feeling down, why not help them by invit-
ing them over for dinner? Take a look at notice boards in your
area. There may be charities or voluntary groups that require
help. Why not give them a hand?

Doing days

Choose between one and six of the tasks shown below, depending
on how you scored on the table on page 137. Tick the ones you
think you want to do (don't worry, you can change them later).

❏   **Walk** Go for a 30-minute walk before or after work, or at
lunchtime. This might serve as a buffer from work, or a decom-
pression chamber for your mind. Walking gives your mind the
space it needs to gain perspective. It helps break the mould so
that you can become more creative. It can catalyse a chain of
events that leads to more insights and, ultimately, strengthens
your willpower. The least it will do is stop you slipping back
into your normal regime.

❑ **Create** Why not enhance your life by creating something new? You could buy a set of watercolours and paint a picture. Or you could use some leftover house paint and use that instead. Why not make an ornament out of clay; you can buy the materials cheaply from an art shop and fire it in your oven. Let your imagination run wild. You could plant some seeds for a window box or buy a mushroom or herb growing kit to produce some of your own food. Why not try baking biscuits, knitting a jumper or making someone a birthday card? Habits kill your creativity, so the best way of freeing yourself is to create something new. It fires up a side of your character that may have been fossilising for years. It doesn't matter what you create. Creativity begets creativity.

❑ **Activity** Try out a new activity or hobby, or perhaps return to one you haven't done for years. The aim is to do something different, not to become an expert. Take it seriously, though, don't just use it to kill time. But don't become competitive either. Try and learn something about yourself. When was the last time you did something that stretched you physically outside of work or made you a more diverse and interesting person? Why not energetically tackle a project that you've been putting off for years, like clearing out the shed or sorting out the attic? It doesn't matter what you choose, but make sure you give it your all; if you feel exhausted afterwards, that's good! You should also notice how fulfilled you feel. You could also try going to your local sports centre to see what activities are on offer. Have you ever considered archery, yoga, t'ai chi, ballroom dancing or fencing, for instance? Or why not borrow some roller blades and try skating? Get your bike out of the shed and go cycling. Or take the kids to the woods and rediscover tree climbing. Remember that the aim is not to take up athletics or an extreme sport (though you can, if you want to), but to discover new and more interesting ways of spending your time. Try it the once. If you don't like it, you don't have to carry on, do you?

'I still don't know how being on the *No Diet Diet* made me lose weight, but it did. On one of my *Do Something Different* days I went a different way to work. It took me about five minutes longer and, to be honest, I didn't see the point of it. But on that journey I spotted a poster for a local choir. I've always loved singing so I gave them a call.

'I now sing with them twice a week and we've even put on performances at local hospitals and old people's homes. I love singing and I've met lots of new people. Getting out and about a bit more and *Doing Something Different* has helped me lose weight. If I hadn't done something different that day, none of this would have happened. I'm glad I've lost weight and I'm equally glad I joined the choir.'

Jan, 49

❏   **Learn** Find out something new about the world. Learn a few unfamiliar words (maybe in a foreign language) or learn how something works – it doesn't need to be a complex, hi-tech gadget, it could be how your heart works, or a car engine. The aim is to discover different ways of interpreting and viewing things. Please remember, if you keep the same knowledge base, you will retain the same ways of thinking. Stretch your mind a bit, you'll be amazed how elastic it is.

❏   **Stand** When you get home from work, or at the end of your normal day, stay upright and don't sit down for at least half an hour. It doesn't matter what you do, just don't sit down. How does it make you feel? Does it give you a different viewpoint? Does it stop you slipping into your old habits? You don't need to rush around, you could do some stretching exercises while you're standing, or dust the ceiling! Remember, it's all about *Doing Something Different*.

❏   **Change** Alter the way you normally do something or the way you look. Sit in the garden and read. If it's not sunny, take a duvet! Or why not try a different hairstyle, clothes or make-up? Dye your hair or paint each of your toenails a different colour. You could also try experimenting with your daily routines by, for example, doing them at different times of the day or in different ways. Arrange to meet a friend for breakfast instead of lunch, or go for a walk with your partner at midnight and look at the stars. Or why not rearrange the furniture in a room you use regularly, or rehang the pictures? Making things look different can make you see things differently too.

Weekly tasks

Phew! Nearly there. All you have to do now is choose two activities from the list of 26 things given below and the preparation for Phase Three is complete. These can be done at any point over the next seven days.

You should choose two things you wouldn't normally do and would not usually feel comfortable doing. Make sure they don't duplicate the things you've already chosen from your Doing list above. It will be easy to do some of them without any effort. But the more effort you put in – and the more different they are from your norm – the better. At this stage, the more you put in, the more weight you'll lose.

NEW THINGS TO TRY	WHEN WILL YOU DO THEM?	TICK WHEN DONE
1. **Music.** Listen to an alternative type of music.		
2. **Clothes.** Wear something totally different.		
3. **Theatre.** Go and see a play.		
4. **Make a list** of your childhood dreams.		
5. **Make** your kids laugh. Don't stop until they're giggling insanely.		
6. **Sing** in the bath.		
7. **Be nice** to someone you do not like.		
8. **Act** as if you don't have a prejudice that you do have.		
9. **Make a list** of your life goals.		
10. **Get up** at a different time.		
11. **Make a list** of the things you do not need.		
12. **Dance** alone for two minutes.		
13. **Make a list** of your goals for next week.		

NEW THINGS TO TRY	WHEN WILL YOU DO THEM?	TICK WHEN DONE
14. **Clean** something you would normally leave untouched.		
15. **Go** and deliberately talk to a neighbour.		
16. **Listen** to a bore. Give him your full attention!		
17. **Say** your own name aloud for one minute.		
18. **List** the good points of your partner.		
19. **Go to bed** one hour earlier.		
20. **Do** something new with the kids.		
21. **Throw** something away that you do not need.		
22. **Estimate** your weight in five years' time.		
23. **Turn** off your mobile phone for a day.		
24. **Learn** a new skill.		
25. **Take up** yoga.		
26. **Practise** being a better listener.		

Step 15   Date

Which type of daily task are you going to do today?
Circle one of the options below.

Doing   People

Which task will you actually do? Tick one of the ones given below.
Remember, more detailed descriptions of the tasks can be found on
pages 138 and 140.

Doing		People	
Walk		Listen	
Create		Ask	
Activity		Give	
Learn		New	
Stand		Find Out	
Change		Help	

Reminder Don't forget the weekly tasks!

Give up the *excuse* habit Try not to make excuses. Be honest with
yourself and others. Face up to the issues you are avoiding.

Step 16   Date

Which type of daily task are you going to do today?
Circle one of the options below.

Doing   People

Which task will you actually do? Tick one of the ones given below.
Remember, more detailed descriptions of the tasks can be found on
pages 138 and 140.

Doing		People	
Walk		Listen	
Create		Ask	
Activity		Give	
Learn		New	
Stand		Find Out	
Change		Help	

Reminder Don't forget the weekly tasks!

Give up the *busy-busy* habit Do you treat life as if it's one big
emergency? Each day build in a little time to relax. Begin training
yourself to respond differently.

Step 17

Date

Which type of daily task are you going to do today?
Circle one of the options below.

Doing   People

Which task will you actually do? Tick one of the ones given below.
Remember, more detailed descriptions of the tasks can be found on
pages 138 and 140.

Doing		People	
Walk		Listen	
Create		Ask	
Activity		Give	
Learn		New	
Stand		Find Out	
Change		Help	

Reminder Don't forget the weekly tasks!

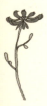

Give up the *fear* habit Don't be daunted by challenges – look at
them as opportunities for growth.

Step 18

18

Date

Which type of daily task are you going to do today?
Circle one of the options below.

Doing   People

Which task will you actually do? Tick one of the ones given below.
Remember, more detailed descriptions of the tasks can be found on
pages 138 and 140.

Doing		People	
Walk		Listen	
Create		Ask	
Activity		Give	
Learn		New	
Stand		Find Out	
Change		Help	

Reminder Don't forget the weekly tasks!

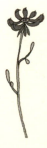

Give up the *talking* habit Most people are good at talking but not
listening. Take time to listen deeply to what someone is saying, don't
interrupt or finish their sentences for them. Talk about them, not you,
and don't expect anything.

Step 19

Date

Which type of daily task are you going to do today?
Circle one of the options below.

Doing   People

Which task will you actually do? Tick one of the ones given below.
Remember, more detailed descriptions of the tasks can be found on
pages 138 and 140.

Doing		People	
Walk		Listen	
Create		Ask	
Activity		Give	
Learn		New	
Stand		Find Out	
Change		Help	

Reminder Don't forget the weekly tasks!

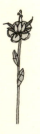

Give up the *blaming* habit Blaming others can become a habit. It's
a way of avoiding responsibility for your own actions. Stop seeing others as responsible for everything that goes wrong. If you make a mistake, don't blame someone else, grab the opportunity to learn from it.

Step 20

Date _____

Which type of daily task are you going to do today?
Circle one of the options below.

Doing   People

Which task will you actually do? Tick one of the ones given below.
Remember, more detailed descriptions of the tasks can be found on
pages 138 and 140.

Doing		People	
Walk		Listen	
Create		Ask	
Activity		Give	
Learn		New	
Stand		Find Out	
Change		Help	

Reminder Don't forget the weekly tasks!

Give up the *taking* habit Try to give or do more than someone
expects of you, and expect nothing in return. Too often we weigh up
what others are doing for us and this leads to negative emotions and
harms relationships.

Step 21

Which type of daily task are you going to do today?
Circle one of the options below.

Doing   People

Which task will you actually do? Tick one of the ones given below.
Remember, more detailed descriptions of the tasks can be found on
pages 138 and 140.

Doing		**People**	
Walk		Listen	
Create		Ask	
Activity		Give	
Learn		New	
Stand		Find Out	
Change		Help	

Reminder Don't forget the weekly tasks!

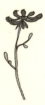

Give up the *past* habit Remember that the past is behind you now.
Stop looking back and living in the past. It is only the present
moment that counts.

KEY POINTS

- You should now be losing a pleasing amount of weight each week. And, around seven days from now, you'll have made so much progress that your weight loss will continue for many weeks and months *after* you've completed the *No Diet Diet* programme.

- You've achieved this remarkable transformation by breaking the habits governing how you interact with other people. You've also broken many more habits that control how you go about 'doing' things in your daily life.

- This has created a virtuous circle that, in the long run, will significantly reduce your weight – and enhance your life.

- The more consistent you've been in breaking your bad habits, the more weight you'll have lost.

CHAPTER NINE

Phase Four: Targeting Transformation

Your net worth to the world is usually determined by what remains after your bad habits are subtracted from your good ones.

Benjamin Franklin

If you're a typical 'non-dieter' your rate of weight loss should have reached cruising speed by now. You should be losing weight at a rate that's best for you. Please accept this as your ideal rate of weight loss and don't try to increase it by too much. Remember, you are not on a diet! We want you to *lose weight permanently*, not just for a month or two. Why not compare the *No Diet Diet* with a food diet (choose any one at random). We reckon that if you were on a food diet instead of ours, that diet would have failed you by now. Nearly three-quarters of people abandon a diet within three weeks. And if you hadn't given up yet on the diet, you'd be racked with food cravings and be close to abandoning it. You'd be tired, irritable and quite possibly depressed. Compare this to how you feel now. Don't you feel happy and full of beans? You've made the correct decision by choosing the *No Diet Diet*.

As we've already said, we've found that people tend to lose around 1 per cent of their body weight *every week* on the *No Diet Diet*, which equates to about 1–2 lb (0.5–1 kg) per week. Some people lose more, others less. But the important thing to remember

153

is how effortless (and fun) the process is. From here onwards, you'll continue losing weight until *your own healthy weight emerges.* This may be in a week or two's time if you were only slightly overweight. Or it could be several months off if you were more overweight. The important thing to remember is that your current rate of weight loss is healthy and sustainable. And it will naturally stabilise at your body's own healthy weight. Our research shows quite clearly that the majority of those who complete Phase Four continue losing weight until they reach their ideal natural weight. So your weight loss will probably continue for many weeks or months after completing the programme. In other words, if you complete Phase Four, *you will never have to go on a food diet again!*

Phase Four is the stage where you finally get to kill off your worst habits and become more flexible. As your old habits melt away, your body will subconsciously continue its shift to a healthier way of living. This will be completely natural and effortless. Phase Four achieves this transformation by targeting key areas of *the way you actually think.*

At this point it's important to remember that there are two types of habit that make up the habitweb (see Chapter Four). Both proximal and distal habits act together to control the three main areas of your life; the way you *think*, the way you *behave* and the way you *do* things. Each habit interlocks and supports all of the rest. The end result is an incredibly tough construction that continuously strengthens and reinforces itself. Of themselves, the habits are weak. But put them together inside the habitweb and they become enormously resilient.

Certain habits kept you fat and these were fixed in place and reinforced by the entire habitweb. Remember that your body doesn't want to be fat. It's only overweight because your bad habits have become welded in place by a habitweb that's become stronger as the years have gone by. In practice, this has meant that it was impossible to make concrete changes to your life by

Roger, 41, has been consistently overweight since his early teens. He was laughed at and bullied at school because of his weight. Since starting the *No Diet Diet* he's lost 2 stone (15.5 kg), and now weighs 11 stone 10 lb (74 kg), which is about right for a man of 5 ft 9 in (1.75 m).

'I'm naturally a bit shy, so, for me, the hardest part of the *No Diet Diet* was Phase Four. I was really worried that I wouldn't be able to change how I behaved. I knew I wanted to, but I wasn't sure if I had what it takes. I decided that I should just try my best and see what happened. The worst part for me was making myself more "fearless". I did this in a small way to start off with. I'm always very worried about speaking in public, even small groups terrify me. So when people were talking at work I'd tell them my opinion. It wasn't easy. I had to force myself. I don't like to be noticed. Everyone seemed to accept my views and carried on talking, and later on they started to ask me how I felt about things.

'I did the same with the other steps in Phase Four. For me taking tiny steps forward was the answer. I really didn't think I could complete Phase Four because of the way I am, but I did it. I'm still too shy and I don't like speaking in public, but at least I've lost weight and I have more confidence in myself.'

tinkering with just a few habits, such as those that govern your diet. This is why diets *always* fail in the end. That's why you have to *Do Something Different* to lose weight. That's why we began in Phase One by tackling the easy habits. As these were broken, we moved further into the core, carefully picking our way through the web. With each step, unravelling the web became easier and easier. Now that we've arrived at the centre we can begin unravelling *the habits that control how you think.*

For most people, how they think and behave is governed by how they thought and behaved in the past. Yes, the way we think is all too often governed by habit too. Buried deep in our subconscious are psychological processes that determine much of what we think, including our attitude to food and exercise. Unfortunately, many of these can become stuck in a rut. Many of our ways of thinking can turn into habits. This is hardly surprising, since the whole of our modern world is geared towards habit-building. The way we work, consume and enjoy our free time is all tightly constrained. Choice is often superficial. This ensures that, day by day, our habits carve deeper tracks. After a while, they cease being superficial habits and become buried deep into our subconscious. And once they are fixed in place they start to govern how we think. As time passes, it becomes increasingly difficult to think independently of our habits. Given that the world is geared towards consuming (especially food), and to making life physically easier, is it any wonder that we're becoming increasingly fat?

'The thing that made a difference for me was shopping at a different supermarket for one of my weekly tasks. I decided to look around carefully and not just pick up the same old things. I bought rice instead of potatoes and found out my family love it. I now experiment with family meals that are much healthier than the ones I cooked before.

'My husband has also taken up cooking, something that amazed me, as he'd never cooked anything more than a bit of toast before. He's lost weight too. Going to a different supermarket was such a small change to make, but it's made a big difference to our lives.'

Helen, 37

You can see that some pretty serious surgery is required on your habitweb. Thankfully, it's almost complete. Phases One, Two and Three began the process. Phase Four completes it and helps you to change your deepest thought processes. Take it from us, they have already started working *for* you rather than *against* you. Once this process is concluded, you'll be infinitely more flexible and adaptable. This will allow you to behave in the way that's best for you. You will no longer be driven by your habits. You will no longer be trapped by your past. You will be absolutely free to make the best decisions possible. In practice, you will no longer be caged inside a vicious cycle of dieting (and getting nowhere). You will lose weight effortlessly, without guilt, anxiety or depression.

You have already proved to yourself that you are capable of change, and that you can break the habits that imprison you, so now it's time to use these new tools to continue losing weight. To kick-start this deeper transformation, each day over the next week we'll ask you to:

- **Behave differently towards a person.**

- **React differently to a situation.**

While you are carrying out these tasks, it's very important that you think about *why* you're doing them. It's vital that you are fully conscious and aware of what you're doing. When you behave automatically and without awareness, your habits are able to take over. That's when diets go wrong and eating problems gain control. If you've got this far, then you are well on the way to changing your deep subconscious. You will have begun adopting a 'slim' way of thinking. Not only does this make life more fun and interesting, but it also brings with it other massive benefits. Weight loss is obviously one, but there are many others. But more of that later.

The feedback we received from the first edition of the *No Diet Diet* revealed that some people found Phase Four more tricky than other parts of the programme. They found it difficult to do the tasks on the days they were supposed to. Some felt that they'd 'failed' the *No Diet Diet* and wondered whether they should give up. If this happens to you, please remember that you have not failed. We have said this many times in the past but it bears repeating: *you do not fail the No Diet Diet*. If you do not manage to do a task on the day you're supposed to, simply pick up where you left off as soon as you can. It really is that straightforward. We'll be reminding you of this as you progress through this chapter.

Our research for this revised edition also revealed that some of the daily tasks weren't always easy for people with busy lives. Some people felt 'rushed' during Phase Four and as a result felt they hadn't put enough effort into doing the tasks. Some said they would have preferred to spend two or even three days completing each step. That way they could fine-tune their habit-breaking and make far more progress. If this happens to you please take extra time to complete each task. We'd love you to do a task each day but don't worry if you can't. Simply spread it over two or three days. Use the first day to get to grips with it and dedicate the second and third days to making substantial progress. Please remember though, the aim is not to achieve perfection but to take a series of small steps forward. If, after three days, you still feel that you haven't made adequate progress, then force yourself to move on to the next task. Then when you have completed Phase Four you can come back and repeat that step before moving on to Phase Five, the lifelong maintenance phase.

Remember the *No Diet Diet* is not an exam or a race where the winner takes all. If, at the end of Step 28, you have learned to love and respect yourself a little more, then you will have achieved something far more precious than weight loss. But rest assured, by the end of Phase Four, 95 per cent of people will have lost a substantial amount of weight.

Before you begin

Each day we'd like you to think carefully for a few minutes about a different *thought-dimension*, such as awareness or fearlessness. A thought-dimension is simply a way of thinking that underlies your behaviour. For example, fearlessness, awareness and emotional intelligence are all different thought-dimensions. Each day we'll give you a different thought-dimension to work with. We'd then like you to apply this thought-dimension to the way you react to a person and a situation you encounter through the day.

This is nowhere near as difficult as it sounds. For example, if the day's dimension is *awareness*, then we'd like you to focus your mind on a person you interact with. We'd like you to make a mental note of such things as the clothes they're wearing, the colour of the flecks in their eyes, the curve of their jawline or the timbre of their voice. On the same day we'd also like you to apply the same thought-dimension to a situation you encounter. For example, if you take the bus to work you might like to make mental notes of the roads you pass by, the sheer variety of people on the bus with you, the colour of the sky, the need for more cycle lanes or perhaps the cheerfulness of the driver (if you're lucky).

Thought-dimensions

The seven key thought-dimensions we'd like you to use over the next week are:

- **Self-responsibility (or accountability)**

- **Awareness**

- **Fearlessness**

- **Balance**

- **Conscience**

- **Emotional intelligence**

- **Social intelligence**

Don't be put off by these terms. They're easy to understand and each one of these dimensions will be explained in detail in due course.

People you'll interact with

Now you need to draw up a list of six people you expect to interact with over the coming week. These might include your partner or spouse, a colleague, a family member, a friend, your boss, or even someone you don't know at all (such as the bus driver). The list is entirely down to you, so why not be imaginative? If you can't come up with six right now, it's OK to come up with just a few and add to them over the next week or so.

Write the people's names here:

1. _____

2. _____

3. _____

4. _____

5. _____

6. _____

Situations you'll encounter

Now you need to draw up a list of situations in which you'd like to apply the different thought-dimensions. They might be situations at home or work that cause you problems or stress. They could also be situations in which things just don't seem to flow as happily as they should do. These might be getting the kids ready for school, driving home from work, a meeting with your boss, queuing at a shop or discussing something with your partner. These will be specific to you. You are the only one who can choose. If you can't come up with six right now, it's OK to come up with just a few and add to them over the next week or so.

Describe the situations here:

1. _____

2. _____

3. _____

4. _____

5. _____

6. _____

What you should do

Each day we want you to take a different thought-dimension and apply it to how you interact with one of the people you named on page 160. You should also apply it to one of the situations you listed.

When interacting with another person
You should think carefully about how you normally behave towards them. Visualise it in your mind. If it helps, write it down. Then work out what changes you plan to make. Your aims are:

• **To behave differently with this person.**

• **Your behaviour should be guided by that day's thought-dimension. This might mean being more extreme, or behaving in the opposite way to how you would normally.**

Again, we can't stress enough that your behaviour should be appropriate to the situation. For example, it might not be a good idea to bed the boss (unless you really want to!) just so you can tick the box.

Situations
You should think carefully about how you normally react in your chosen situation. Visualise it clearly in your mind. Write it down, if it helps. Then work out how you'll deal with the situation this time. Your aims are:

• **To react differently to how you would normally.**

• **Your behaviour should be guided by that day's dimension. This might mean reacting in the opposite way to what your habit-driven reflexes are demanding. Or perhaps you should be more extreme than normal. Only you can decide.**

Remember, the idea is to *Do Something Different*, so don't choose the same person or situation each day.

Step 22   Date

Today's thought-dimension is:

Self-responsibility

Self-responsibility is the degree to which you accept personal accountability for yourself. It means not blaming others for your misfortune, or for the situation in which you find yourself. It's your motivator, self-limiter and mission-setter *so use it to the full*.

Your task for today is to change the way you behave so you can enhance your *self-responsibility*. This might mean not doing something you normally do, or it might mean taking an entirely new course of action. It might also mean:

- **Not making excuses for your failings. For example, if you're late for a drink with a friend, why not be honest? Don't blame the bus or the traffic, admit that it's your fault.**

- **Not blaming other people when things go wrong. Again, be honest with yourself. Admit your own failings in the matter, it's too easy – and sometimes a 'cop out' – to blame others.**

- **If you drive to work, why not be more considerate to pedestrians and stop at every zebra crossing where you see someone waiting? Or perhaps allow more cars to pull out from side roads, give cyclists a wider berth or give a bus the chance to leave its stop? For a change, take public transport.**

- **If you live with your partner, why not make sure you do only your share of the housework, cooking and gardening – and no more. If you're normally a bit slack about these things, why not take the initiative for a change?**

- Take responsibility for your share of global warming and set the thermostat on your central heating one degree lower. You can always put an extra T-shirt or jumper on. While you're at it, why not plant a tree to soak up some carbon dioxide? You could even join a local tree-planting group or set one up with some friends. Failing that, contact www.co2balance.com

- If you've got into the habit of dropping litter, today would be a good day to stop. Why not go one step further and pick up a piece of litter blowing down the street?

- If there's someone you don't get along with, stop expecting them to change and instead alter the way you act towards them. You'll be surprised by the result.

- Do you blame your parents for the failings in your own life? Give them a break and realise that you are the person YOU created.

- Doing something to change a situation, even if the impact you make is only small. For example, you might like to help two friends or family members settle a dispute.

- Making your position known on an issue and taking a stand. Whether this concerns a war in the Middle East, an increasingly unreasonable colleague or the closure of a local school, why not politely but firmly make your views heard?

- Ceasing to see other people or external factors as being the cause of your predicament. You are in the present situation largely because of the decisions you made in the past. Accept it, learn from it, and move on.

- Taking the next step towards a goal and stopping waiting for others to act. Why not take the lead at work and organise a recycling bin or offer to air a grievance on behalf of your colleagues? If you want an extra special or adventurous holi-day, why not research the options now and take the first step towards putting your plans into action?

- **Not believing in fate, luck or your horoscope – remember, you make your own destiny.**

Now we're going to put self-responsibility into action so choose a person from the list you drew up earlier (the one on page 160).

Person chosen _____

Putting it into practice

Decide what you are going to try today with this person to enhance your self-responsibility. For example, you might say to yourself, 'I won't say "yes" to my colleague today every time he asks me to do something for him and then moan to myself about how much I've got to do. I'll either do it without moaning, or I'll refuse politely.' Write below what you have decided to do:

_____

_____

_____

_____

_____

_____

Next, we're going to put self-responsibility into action by using it in one of the situations from the list you drew up earlier (the one on page 161).

Situation chosen _____

Putting it into practice

Decide how you are going to employ your self-responsiblity today. For example, you might say to yourself, 'I'll not read my horoscope today. I'll write my own and then I can make sure it happens'. Write below what you have decided to do.

_____

_____

_____

_____

_____

_____

How did you do?

You should now reflect on what you did, the effect it had, and any changes you noticed. To help you, here are a few questions you might like to consider:

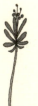

*   **How did other people react to your enhanced self-responsibility?**

*   **How did it make you feel?**

*   **Can you see any other benefits to acting this way?**

Make notes here:

_____

_____

_____

_____

_____

_____

_____

_____

_____

_____

Step 23   **Date**

Today's thought-dimension is:

Awareness

Remember, if you've missed a day, just pick up where you left off. You don't fail the *No Diet Diet*!

If you don't feel you've made enough progress today, why not repeat this step tomorrow? Don't punish yourself though – the aim .is to take small steps forward every day.

Awareness is being conscious of your emotional state and the impact you have on others. See it as an impartial extra eye that constantly keeps a lookout for you and on everything that goes on around you.

Today you should try increasing and enhancing your awareness. You should begin by listing ten new things that you notice about a person chosen from the list you drew up earlier (the one on page 160). This could include their habits, behaviour and attitudes, and the way they respond to you. You should try and include some physical features too. Also today you should list ten new things that you have noticed or learnt about your everyday environment.

Please remember that the aim of Step 23 is not to behave differently, although you may need to do something different, but to find out something new.

To help build your awareness, here are a few examples of the sort of things that you might like to focus your attention on before you do today's tasks. You could pick a few from this list and focus your attention on them. The more you fine-tune your awareness, the better you'll become at breaking your bad habits. Why not try:

• **Listening to the words of a song.**

- Learning something new about a person who is not important to you but with whom you come into contact. For example, the driver of the bus you catch each morning or the postman.

- Listening out for sounds that you're not normally aware of. This could be anything from birdsong to the sound of the central heating firing up.

- Focusing your attention on something you do automatically, such as cleaning your teeth or driving your car.

- Considering the effect your behaviour has on other people. Watch carefully how people react to you.

- Paying attention to something you wouldn't normally notice, such as the texture of the paper your favourite magazine is printed on or the sweet smell of grass.

- Focusing in more detail on one of your regular tasks at work.

- Becoming more attuned to the things that you normally pass by without noticing.

- Focusing your attention on all aspects of the places you visit. Notice the smells, colours, textures and even the tastes of everywhere you go.

To further enhance your awareness you might like to try:

- Asking someone to give you feedback about something you said or did.

- Using a different form of transport to make a regular journey. You could even try walking or cycling there.

- Discovering something new about your street.

- Staying a little longer. This could be at work, at home, or maybe you could linger at the bus stop or station. How does it feel?

- **Travelling to a familiar place, such as work or a friend's house, by a different route.**

- **Reading a different section of the newspaper.**

- **Getting up 15 minutes earlier and spending the time looking around your house or flat.**

Now we're going to put your heightened awareness into action, so choose a person from the list you drew up earlier (on page 160). Use your awareness to learn more about this person, how they think, feel, behave and live their life. This may seem a little odd at first, but focusing on an individual in this way helps you break the habit of always seeing them in the same light. Very soon you'll look at everyone afresh and your whole life will suddenly become more interesting. No longer will you 'see through a glass, darkly'. Awareness is a key skill in conscious behaviour – when you are operating with awareness, habits cannot keep their grip on you.

Person chosen _____

What have you become aware of?

List below ten new things of which you have become aware. For example, 'Geoff always gives excuses' or 'Sheila always looks perky after she's said something at a meeting'.

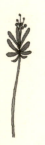

1. _____

2. _____

3. _____

4. _____

5. _____

6. _____

7. _____

8. _____

9. _____

10. _____

Environment chosen

This could be your home, workplace or a nearby park. The location doesn't matter, but you might as well be creative and enjoy yourself.

_____

What have you become aware of?

List below ten new things of which you have become aware. For example, 'The daffodils in the park are about to flower' or 'There is a lot of litter around'.

1. _____

2. _____

3. _____

4. _____

5. _____

6. _____

7. _____

8. _____

9. _____

10. _____

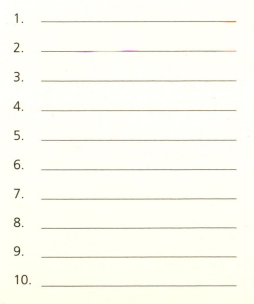

How did you do?

You now need to reflect on what you did. To help you, here are a few questions you might like to consider:

- **How did other people react to your enhanced awareness?**

- **How did it make you feel?**

- **Have you lacked awareness in the past and operated wearing blinkers?**

- **What else might you have been missing?**

- **Can you see any other benefits to acting this way?**

Make notes here:

_____

_____

_____

_____

_____

_____

Remember, awareness is the enemy of habits and an important step on the way to acting flexibly and maintaining your weight loss.

Step 24   Date

Today's thought-dimension is:

Balance

Balance involves making sure every aspect of your life receives its appropriate share of care and attention. The most important parts of your life, such as relationships, should obviously be given the most attention. The least important parts should receive proportionately less attention. Balance is the process of 'divvying up' your attention to maximise life's rewards. Get it wrong, and life will be infinitely less satisfying, or may even fall apart completely.

Today you'll begin tweaking your life to achieve a better balance. It's worth remembering that you can do this in one of two ways (or a mixture of both). Firstly, you can act to put more or less effort into a relationship or situation. Or secondly, you can change how you view a relationship or situation. For example, the exercises on the following page may make you realise how much – or how little – you care for a person in your life. You can then act to change the level of effort you put into that relationship. Alternatively, you can increase or decrease the importance you attach to that person. If you follow the former course, you act, whereas if you adopt the latter course, you change your view. Only you can decide what to do.

Over the following few pages you'll be encouraged to think and behave in ways that enhance balance. But remember, you are the best judge of where the point of balance lies. Depending on many competing interests, you may feel, for example, that you want temporarily to put your career before relationships (though this can, in the long run, be a dangerous strategy). You are the best judge of where the balance points lie.

To enhance balance, you might like to try:

- **Evaluating the importance of everything you do, from shopping through to work and your pastimes. Is each and everything you do worth the effort?**

- **Evaluating the importance of all the people with whom you come into contact. You should rate the amount of satisfaction you gain from each of them and the effort you put into maintaining the relationship. For example, if you put a lot of effort into maintaining a friendship with someone but get little in return, perhaps you should reconsider their importance to you and how much you're willing to give.**

Other points to ponder include:

- **Are you putting enough effort into your most important relationships? British workers spend on average 49 minutes per day checking their emails and 25 minutes a day playing with their kids. Are these people, in your opinion, leading balanced lives?**

- **Should you be spending more time with your partner, friends or children?**

- **Are you spending too much time at work?**

- **Why are you not doing precisely what you want to do right now – *this minute*!**

- **Is it time to take a break from someone or from a difficult situation in which you find yourself?**

- **Why not show someone how special they are to you? You could phone them, write to them, buy them a little gift or go out for a coffee with them.**

- **Why are you not spending more time doing the things you want to do and less time doing the things you don't want to do?**

- **Are you surrounded by possessions that mean nothing to you? If you are, why do you still have them? Remember, possessions possess. Enjoy getting rid of them rather than acquiring them.**

- **Why not put less effort into poor relationships that have little to offer you?**

- **Why not re-establish a lost friendship that once meant a lot to you?**

Now we're going to kick-start your quest for balance. Firstly, choose a person who is important to you from the list you drew up earlier on page 160. Now consider how much effort you're putting into that relationship. Is it too much or too little? Once you've decided your answer, you should then change the amount of effort you put in to reflect the relationship's importance to you. And afterwards see what happens to your level of satisfaction.

Person chosen _____

Putting it into practice

Are you going to put in more or less effort? How specifically will you do this? For example, will you call them more or less often, go out with them more frequently or less? (Remember, you can either change the way you behave or alter the way you view this person.)

Write what you plan to do here. For example, you might write, 'I will carry on meeting Jane once a week, but I'll suggest we take it in turns to meet near each other's home, rather than me always going over to her.'

_____

_____

_____

_____

_____

_____

Now we're going to enhance your balance by using it in one of the situations from the list you drew up earlier on page 161.

Situation chosen _____

Putting it into practice

How are you going to enhance your balance today? Remember, you can either change your behaviour or change the way you view the situation.

Write what you plan to do here. For example, you might write, 'I'll set a time limit on how long I spend doing the cleaning at the weekend and do something with the kids with the extra time.'

_____

_____

_____

_____

_____

_____

_____

How did you do?

You now need to reflect on what you did, the effect it had, and any changes you noticed. To help you, here are a few questions you might like to consider:

- **How did other people react to your enhanced sense of balance?**

- **How did it make you feel?**

- **Have you lacked balance in the past and operated wearing blinkers?**

- **Have you got genuine balance in your life now or could you work on it a little more?**

Make notes here:

_____

_____

_____

_____

_____

_____

_____

_____

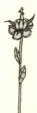

Step 25

Date

Today's thought-dimension is:

Fearlessness

Remember, if you've missed a day, just pick up where you left off. You don't fail the *No Diet Diet*!

If you don't feel you've made enough progress today, why not repeat this step tomorrow? Don't punish yourself though – the aim is to take small steps forward every day.

Firstly, we'd like to reassure you. To get through today, you won't need to become a lion-tamer, go paragliding off a mountain or canoe across the Atlantic (unless you want to, of course).

To be fearless means acting without nervousness or trepidation. It means facing the unknown with the same bravado as the mundane. Fearlessness is a willingness to go outside your comfort zone. Today's task is to enhance your fearlessness by doing things that you would normally avoid because they make you feel uncomfortable. Fearlessness is a great habit-slayer and very empowering. Once you've felt fear and carried on regardless, you'll be able to achieve anything you want in life.

To behave fearlessly today, you'll need to put yourself in a situation that causes you anxiety. You'll also need to interact with a person who causes you fear. The fear you experience need not be great, and if you are genuinely frightened, please find something a little less extreme! The aim is to push the boundaries, to get you to operate outside your comfort zone and to face up to what you've been avoiding, not to paralyse you with fright.

In practice, you can encourage fearlessness by, for example:

- Taking action over something you've been worrying about. What's worrying you most at this precise moment? Why not take action – any action – right now? Making a decision will move you in the right direction because concrete action conquers fear. Doing nothing allows fear to control you.

- Tackling a phobia, such as speaking in public or a fear of spiders.

- Saying 'no' to someone who takes advantage of you or who expects too much of you.

- Asking for what you want and not being afraid of looking foolish. This could be in bed with your partner or over an issue at work.

- Doing something you've put off for ages because of your fears. Perhaps you've got a financial problem you're not facing? Tell somebody that you need help even if you don't know what to do. Phone a helpline or an advisory service. The Citizens Advice Bureau could well end up being the answer to your prayers.

- Doing something to take you out of your comfort zone in an area that's important to you. For example, maybe you've put off going to the dentist for a check-up – now's the time to make an appointment.

- Talking about a difficult subject with someone. This could be about anything that scares you or makes you feel uncomfortable. Take the bull by the horns and say, 'I need to talk to you about X, would now be a good time?'

- Buddying up with someone to help you get over your fear. Admitting your fears is nothing to be ashamed of and you might be surprised at how supportive others are. So, ask a friend to go to the bank manager with you, or ask a relative to accompany you to see a consultant.

Now you need to put fearlessness into action, so choose a person from the list you drew up earlier on page 160.

Person chosen _____

Putting it into practice

Decide what you are going to try with this person today that will make you more fearless. You might, for example, say to yourself, 'I'll stop ignoring Peter's sexual innuendoes and warn him privately that if he does it again I'll report him to his boss and the personnel department.' Write below what you have decided to do:

_____

_____

_____

_____

_____

Now you can put fearlessness into practice in one of the situations on the list you drew up earlier on page 161. If there isn't a situation on the list that causes you fear, try and think of one now and use this one instead.

Situation chosen _____

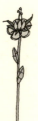

Putting it into practice

Decide how you are going to behave fearlessly in the situation you've chosen. For example, you might say to yourself, 'The next time a spider is in the bath I'll catch it and release it outside. I'll remind myself that spiders catch insects and flies' or 'I will phone someone I know who might offer me a better job and ask if I can send them my CV.' Write below what you've decided to do:

_____

_____

_____

_____

_____

_____

How did you do?

Now you need to reflect on what you did and the effect it had. To help you, here are a few questions you might like to consider:

- **How did it make you feel? (Be more specific than 'it frightened me'.)**

- **How did other people react to your enhanced fearlessness?**

- **Do you now feel more in control of your life?**

- **Can you see any other benefits to facing up to your fears?**

- **Have you started to extend the boundaries of your comfort zone?**

- **Have you lacked fearlessness in the past?**

- **How might this have affected your life?**

Make notes here:

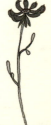

_____

_____

_____

Sarah, 26, kept a diary of her experiences with the *No Diet Diet*. She quickly lost a substantial amount of weight but admits that some parts of the programme were very tough going. She wrote:

'I was terrified of doing Step 25 because I had to dwell on fearlessness and doing things that scared me. So I decided to be more open about being a Christian with people I don't know. I fell at the first hurdle when I had a meeting with a potential supplier. I had intended to slip into conversation that I go to church but somehow I couldn't manage it. I could even feel myself blushing and stuttering every time I intended to mention it.

'Why did I worry about it? I now realise that fear is an emotion I feel far too much of the time. I really want to feel it less, or – to put it a better way – overcome it more.

'Then I gave myself a second task: I planned to stand around not doing anything at a networking event, even though it made me look like a total Billy no-mates. After the event I could hear an internal dialogue going on; my inner voice shouting at me for damaging my career, etc. Still, I'd taken a small step down the road to fearlessness.

'Then – rather too spookily for my liking – I had a chance encounter in Oxford Street with an ex-boyfriend I've never quite got over. I could swear my heart stopped when I saw him in the distance. I did my best to look away but couldn't manage it. I thought to myself, in a very Paxman tone of voice: "Oh, COME OFF IT. I've got to get over this!"

'I realised that I might not get over him completely in one day but I could take a small step forward. So I hid behind a bus shelter and looked round it very, very slowly, cartoon style, until I could just see him from a distance. I stared for a few seconds and scampered off into the crowd! A small step forward!

'The thing I like most about the *No Diet Diet* is that the book repeats quite often that you can't fail it. If something's too hard for you, you just have to take smaller steps, until you achieve them, and then build up to bigger things in increments. The point is not to measure your progress but just to try, and enjoy the feeling you get when you succeed.'

Step 26   **Date**

Today's thought-dimension is:

Conscience

Conscience is differentiating right from wrong and then acting on it. Conscience adds the personal moral and ethical dimension to your life. Your conscience should be listened to in all contexts, regardless of whether it's convenient to do so or not.

With this in mind, today's task is to listen to and apply what your conscience dictates at all times. This will increase the power of your conscience and help you achieve what you want, as well as making life a little better for those around you. Today's task doesn't require you to change your morals or ethics in any way – it's designed to make sure that you apply them in whatever you do. This might mean not doing something you would normally do, or it might mean taking an entirely new course of action. Before you start today's main tasks, draw up a list of five core principles you want to live your life by. These might be values you aspire to but sometimes (or often) fail to achieve. They could include kindness, patience, honesty, moderation, faithfulness, hard work, love, respect, regular prayer, being a good friend, good neighbourliness, caring for animals, etc. The aim of this list is to identify the values that lie closest to your heart. Make a copy of this list and keep it with you throughout today.

Write your five core values here:

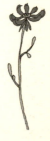

_____

_____

_____

_____

_____

Now spend today without violating *any* of your values in any way. For example, it might mean:

- **Making sure that you do not compromise yourself for short-term gain. Do you really need to tell a lie when honesty will do?**

- **Doing unto others as you would be done unto yourself.**

- **Treating someone with more respect. This could be someone you phone, such as a person in a bank call centre, or a person you meet, such as the new girlfriend of an ex-partner.**

- **Avoiding greed. Consuming more than you need is a habit that leads to unhappiness (and huge credit card bills). So spend the day without lusting after such little extravagancies as new shoes, a facial or even visiting a café on the way home from work.**

- **Avoiding mental or physical laziness. Life is for living and you're only here once. Why aren't you making the most of every precious moment?**

- **Avoiding conflict. Petty battles consume vast amounts of energy, energy that you could be using to improve your life and those of the people around you. Are you trapped by the habit of arguing with your mother, partner or a once-close friend? Today is the day to break this habit by refusing to engage in any form of conflict.**

- **Flee envy and jealousy. It might be pleasant to own a new car like one of your workmates, move into the bigger flat next door, or go on regular spending sprees, but will they make you truly happy? Envy and jealousy can reinforce incredibly powerful habits. Avoid them like the plague today!**

- **Not using a stereotype to judge other people. Drop your prejudices. They're bad for you, bad for the people you're prejudiced against, and bad for society!**

- **Treating all the people you meet equally. This involves being courteous, kind and reasonable. It also involves being firm, but reasonable, if the situation demands it.**

- **When making a decision, ask yourself what is the RIGHT thing to do. Doing the right thing is what should guide your action, rather than what you usually do or what others expect you to do.**

- **Not being tempted to do something you know is wrong. Do you really need to raid the office stationery cupboard or make so many private calls from work?**

  Your next step is to apply your conscience in all its glory, so choose a person from the list you drew up earlier on page 160. Remember, this person is the focus of your task but you should still try and apply your core values to every person you meet.

  Person chosen _____

Putting it into practice

Decide what you will do to enhance your conscience. For example, you might say to yourself, 'I won't join in with Ruth today when she starts to gossip about Alex. I'll say that Alex's behaviour is her own business and I won't be drawn into constantly criticising her.' Write below what you have decided to do. But remember – you should try to apply your core values to every person you meet:

_____

_____

_____

_____

_____

Now we're going to enhance your conscience by applying it in one of the situations from the list you drew up earlier on page 161.

Situation chosen _____

Putting it into practice

Decide how you are going to apply your conscience today. For example, you might say to yourself, 'If my computer crashes, I will not lose my temper with the IT support people. I'll try to understand that they did not make my computer crash, it's an accident.' Write below what you've decided to do but remember to apply your core values in all situations today.

_____

_____

_____

_____

_____

_____

_____

_____

_____

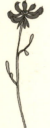

How did you do?

Now you need to reflect on what you did and the effect it had. To help you, here are a few questions you might like to consider:

- **How did other people react to your enhanced conscience?**
- **How did it make you feel?**

- **Have you lacked conscience in the past?**

- **What have you missed as a result?**

- **What are the long-term benefits of acting this way?**

Make notes here:

_____

_____

_____

_____

_____

_____

_____

_____

_____

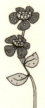

Step 27   **Date**

Today's thought-dimension is:

Emotional intelligence

Emotional intelligence is the ability to recognise your own emotions and those of the people around you. It is also the capacity to use your emotions and those of others to help rather than hinder you. See it as your emotional thermometer and manager.

Today's task is to increase your emotional intelligence. The idea is to re-tune your mind so that you can spot your emotions before they overwhelm you. This is not cold-hearted or calculating, it's simply a way of making sure that your emotions don't run away with you. It will allow you to experience the full range of emotions, not to remain stuck in the rut of just one or two. Finely tuning your emotional intelligence will help you achieve just this.

Many people's habits cage them and force them to experience only a narrow range of emotions, such as anger and unhappiness. Habitual dieters are especially trapped in a narrow range of emotions; anxiety, unhappiness and guilt are all the inevitable end-result of dieting. After a while, of course, these negative emotions become so ingrained and habitual that happiness and balance become just a distant memory. Only by breaking free of these can you begin to really experience life.

A high degree of emotional intelligence puts you back in the driving seat. Emotions have a very important role to play – they make life worth living for a start – but if they seize control of your mind then they can wreck your happiness.

Today you will change the way you think and behave to enhance your emotional intelligence. You might do this by:

- Labelling emotions. Try and define the emotions that other people feel when they are around you and react accordingly. And stop reacting solely to what they say and do. Look beyond their words for deeper meanings. Don't take people literally, stop and consider what they might feel, not just what they say.

- Take the emotion out of a situation. When you feel an emotion building up inside you, don't just react, do what's best. Think! Consider whether your feeling is justified, or if there could be an alternative explanation to which you could react differently – with a different emotion.

- In a situation, or with a person, choose an alternative way of feeling. A good way of doing this is to change how you respond. If, for example, you feel angry about someone's opinion, don't scowl at them, smile instead. Pretty soon you'll feel sorry for them being so narrow-minded. Remember, *Do Something Different*! This might not be easy at first, but you've already proved that you're capable of change.

- When you meet with someone, imagine you are in the other person's shoes and react accordingly. Forget your own nervousness at a first encounter and consider how ill-at-ease the other person might be feeling.

- Express your emotions, but only when it won't do any harm – don't just explode at one of your colleagues or family members. Only express negative emotions after careful consideration. Ask yourself whether you express your positive emotions enough; tell someone when you are happy or excited about something.

- Instead of being naturally defensive, take a more positive stance or loosen up. For example, it's OK to admit when you're feeling nervous, even if you're a big boss. Admitting to these emotions simply lets other people know that you are human.

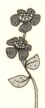

Remember, if you've missed a day, just pick up where you left off. You don't fail the *No Diet Diet*!

Now we're going to put emotional intelligence into action. Firstly, you should focus on yourself to hone your skills. Then you can move on to a person chosen from the list you drew up earlier on page 160. So let's start with you. What are you going to do today that will enhance your emotional intelligence? (You may wish to choose an example from the list on page 189 – but please be creative!) You might, for example, say to yourself, 'I'll keep an eye on my emotions. I'll try not to "just react" or fly off the handle. I'll label them and see if I can try to feel a different emotion instead.' Write down what you plan to do here:

_____

_____

_____

_____

_____

Now you need to increase your emotional intelligence by using it in a real-life situation with another person chosen from the list you drew up on page 160.

Person chosen _____

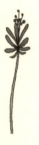

Putting it into practice

How will you use your emotional intelligence to enhance your dealings with this person? You might, for example, say to yourself, 'I'll try to stop myself being defensive in today's team meeting with Curtis. I'm new, so they can't expect me to know everything straightaway. If necessary, I'll remind them of this. I'll see if I can spot Curtis's emotional responses and see how they change when I become less defensive.' Write down what you plan to do here:

_____

_____

_____

_____

_____

_____

> If you don't feel you've made enough progress today, why not repeat this step tomorrow? Don't punish yourself though – the aim is to take small steps forward every day.

How did you do?

Now you should reflect on what you did. To help you, here are a few questions you might like to consider:

- **How did it make you feel?**

- **Were you able to gain an insight into how your interactions might be driven by emotions – both your own and others'?**

- **How did other people react to your enhanced emotional intelligence?**

- **Have you lacked emotional intelligence in the past and operated wearing blinkers?**

- **What else might you have been missing?**

- **Can you see any benefits in improving your emotional intelligence?**

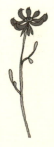

Make notes here:

_____

_____

_____

_____

_____

_____

Jackie, 31, decided to fine-tune her emotional intelligence by noticing and naming the emotions she felt when she met a group of friends she hadn't seen in many years. She also went further than was strictly necessary by spotting and writing down the emotions of everyone else she met through the day.

'I'm terrible at dealing with emotion. I'm not too bad at enjoying myself but as soon as I experience an emotion I don't like such as sadness or grief, I try to stifle it and hope it never comes back. I do the same with other people. If somebody else is upset or frightened, I do my best to make it go away, even if it means doing something totally inappropriate like cracking a joke at a funeral.

'So the "emotional intelligence" task was a real challenge for me. I quickly realised that most of the emotions I feel I can't actually name. As soon as I started, I realised I was pulling my finger out of a crack in an enormous dam. Life suddenly became a lot more raw. In some ways it was fun but in others it was a little unsettling. I decided to spend several days on this task. Although it's still something I need to work on, I feel better about expressing my emotions and I'm more confident overall.'

Step 28

Date

Today's thought-dimension is:

Social intelligence

Social intelligence is helping others and society in general. See it as a way of expressing your values in a positive and practical way.

A highly attuned sense of social intelligence helps create a feeling of 'warmth' inside you, which chases away negative emotions. These negative emotions can be especially resilient habits that are particularly difficult to break. Enhancing social intelligence is a powerful weapon against these bad habits. And, as you know, bad habits make you fat! Break 'em and you'll lose weight.

Today's task is to increase your social intelligence in a selfless way. Examples might be:

- **Helping a person out. If someone needs help, why not lend a hand? It might mean helping a relative move house or helping a friend prepare for a party or barbeque.**

- **Ethical purchasing. When shopping, look out for things that accord with your values, such as Fair Trade coffee or other goods. At Christmas, make sure the cards you buy benefit a charity. Look in charity shops for other things you'd routinely buy, for example pens, candles or small presents. Why not buy from small shops so that ordinary people rather than big businesses get the benefit of your money?**

- Fine-tune your social intelligence at work. Why not bring in a few potted plants or flowers to brighten the office? Why not make the tea or coffee (even if it isn't your turn)? Make a real effort to help an 'outsider' fit into the workplace. This could be a new recruit or someone who isn't generally liked by your workmates.

- Learn something about a minority group or a 'cause'. Search out fund-raising events that aim to raise money for disadvantaged or sick people. Consider supporting them or even taking part in one of their fund-raising events, such as a sponsored walk.

- Do something for your local community (even if it is just picking up some litter). There's probably somewhere you can recycle old shoes, mobile phones, clothes and even computers.

- Plant a tree on some waste ground. And, while you're at it, why not sprinkle some wildflower seeds around too.

* If you are a manager, today might be a good day to encourage your workers to work together more as a team. Ask them collectively how the workplace could be improved and how it could be run more effectively. Have you considered having a team outing once a month? This could be to the cinema, pub or somewhere unexpected such as the theatre. If you don't have a suitable place, why not establish a 'suggestion box' with prizes for the best ideas? And don't just listen – do your best to act.

- Give something back to society without thought of immediate gain. Think about becoming a volunteer in your spare time, just an hour or two a week could really make a difference.

- **Join an environmental or animal welfare group and volunteer your services. There are plenty out there and they constantly need help. Why not phone them and see?**

- **Watch how people do their jobs and how you fit into the bigger picture. You have a role – if you didn't, they wouldn't be paying your wages. Are you happy or do you want to progress up the career ladder? If you do, why not think – or ask your boss – how you can go about this?**

- **Care a little more about something close to your social values. Choose the issue closest to your heart and learn as much as you can about it.**

Now you need to put your social intelligence into action, so choose a person from the list you drew up earlier on page 160.

Person chosen _____

Putting it into practice

Decide what you are going to try today with this person to enhance your social intelligence. For example, you might say to yourself, 'I'll encourage the kids to pick up some litter on the way to school and make them aware of an environmental issue' or 'I'll leave all the extra apples from my tree at the front gate with a sign asking people to help themselves.' Write below what you plan to do:

_____

_____

_____

_____

_____

_____

Next you're going to put social intelligence into action by using it in one of the situations from the list you drew up earlier on page 161.

Situation chosen _____

Putting it into practice

How are you going to employ your social intelligence today? You might, for example, say to yourself, 'Tonight when I go shopping I'll buy organic or Fair Trade goods wherever I can' or 'I'll take everything I can to the recycling bins down the road (on foot so I don't waste petrol) rather than throwing it out.' Write what you plan to do below:

_____

_____

_____

_____

_____

_____

_____

How did you do?

Now you need to reflect on what you did. To help you, here are a few questions you might like to consider:

- **How did other people react to your enhanced social intelligence?**

- **How did it make you feel?**

- **Have you lacked social intelligence in the past?**

- **What else might you have been missing?**

- **Is this an area of your life you could develop more?**

- **Can you see any other benefits to acting this way?**

Make notes here:

_____

_____

_____

_____

_____

_____

_____

_____

KEY POINTS

- You've done it! You have successfully broken most, if not all, of the bad habits that have kept you over-weight for years.

- Our research shows that you should have lost around 7–9 lb (3–4 kg) since you started the *No Diet Diet.*

- Phase Four targeted the habits that govern how you think. Since the start of the *No Diet Diet* you have successfully targeted the bad habits that govern how you do things, how you behave and how you think. These habits effectively imprisoned you and preven-ted you from fulfilling your dream of losing weight.

- Your actual degree of weight loss reflects how well you managed to break your most intransigent bad habits.

- One thing is for certain, you should no longer be driv-en by your habits or trapped by your past. You are no longer caged inside a vicious cycle of dieting and failure.

- Your weight should continue to decline for many more weeks and months until your ideal healthy weight emerges. But this weight loss may eventually stall unless you embed your progress. Phase Five of the programme is designed to do this.

CHAPTER TEN

Phase Five: Getting What You Want – Your Ideal Weight

Habit is habit and not to be flung out of the window by any man, but coaxed downstairs a step at a time.

Mark Twain

We've got some great news for you. You're now an accomplished 'non-dieter'. You'll never need to go on a diet again! You've reached the point where your weight will continue to decline of its own accord until your ideal healthy figure emerges. Not for you are hunger pangs, anxiety and dieting depression. We hope that you'll now agree, the secret to losing weight is ditching the diet habit.

At this point in a conventional diet book, the authors would be giving you stern warnings about the dangers of slipping back into your old weight-gaining ways. They'd gently break the news to you that you'd have to stay on the diet for the rest of your life. As an occasional treat you'd be allowed an extra mouthful of pumpkin seeds, or perhaps a small, dry, low-carb biscuit. This would be your life from this point onwards. No wonder dieting makes you depressed.

As you know, the *No Diet Diet* doesn't make you anxious, depressed or induce irresistible food cravings. As a result, we won't need to warn you about backsliding. Nor will we try and sell you a cookbook. The *No Diet Diet* is the only weight-loss programme you'll ever need.

What surprises people most about the *No Diet Diet* is that it continues to work long after they've completed the initial 28-step programme. In fact, this is when it really comes into its own. With the *No Diet Diet*, the weight loss you have achieved so far is only the beginning. This is because you've succeeded in breaking a critical mass of habits. This gives your willpower the breathing space it needs to help you achieve the weight loss you crave. Your mind is once again in control, not your habits. You've adopted the mind-set of the slim. This ensures that you'll gradually lose weight until your body's own healthy weight emerges. Phase Five enhances this process and fine-tunes your habit-breaking. But more of that in a moment.

Weight loss

If our clients and clinical trials are any guide, you should have lost around 8 lb (3.5 kg) in weight by now. The actual degree of weight loss reflects how well you managed to break your most intransigent bad habits. Rest assured, whether you've lost more or less fat than average, your weight will almost certainly carry on diminishing. Some people's habits are easier to break than others. In practice, this means that weight loss differs from person to person. Some people make huge strides with the *No Diet Diet*. Others have to work a little harder at habit-breaking to get the same result. So please remember, you won't fail the *No Diet Diet*!

Beth, one of our clients, has in many ways become a typical 'non-dieter'. By the time she was 35 she'd spent the best part of the previous 15 years yo-yo dieting. And the result? At 5 ft 5 in (1.65 m) she weighed 12 stone 7 lb (79.5 kg) – around 32 lb (14.5 kg) more than the ideal. Clearly, every diet she'd tried had failed her. From low-calorie to high-fibre, from low-carb to low-fat, every single weight-loss regime Beth had tried had simply ensured she'd gained more weight in the long run.

At the end of Phase Four of the *No Diet Diet* Beth was delighted. She'd lost 4 lb (2 kg) – hardly a resounding success you might think. After all, she was right at the bottom of the weight-loss range promised by the *No Diet Diet*. But Beth was still very pleased with herself.

'I'd given up on dieting and on myself,' she told us. 'But I decided to give the *No Diet Diet* a go. I thought it sounded easy and fun and it couldn't do any harm. I expected to fail, but I lost weight and I'm still losing weight. That's important to me. It gives me hope. I know that I can become slim again. It may take me a lot longer than many people who do the *No Diet Diet*, but I know that I can do it. To be my ideal weight, I think will take me another six months. What the hell! Smelling flowers in the park, taking a different route to work and deepening my relationship with my partner are hardly difficult things to do. If I carry on losing 1 lb (0.5 kg) a week doing things like that I'll be more than delighted!'

Three months after talking to us, Beth was still slowly but surely losing weight. She'd lost 16 lb (7.2 kg) by the time spring came. By the time she went on her summer holiday she'd lost 21 lb (9.5 kg).

'For the first time in at least a decade I didn't look like a beached whale on my holidays!' she told us. 'I'd still like to lose another 10–15 lb (6–7 kg). It'll take me another few months, but I can wait.'

Beth is consistently losing weight and she knows that soon enough she'll have the figure she wants. We hope that your experiences of the *No Diet Diet* are even better than Beth's. It may seem odd to you that she could be so happy. After all, she performed right at the bottom of the weight-loss range typically achieved by our 'non-dieters'. This highlights another crucial difference between the *No Diet Diet* and food-based diets: it makes you happy and improves your self-esteem. She's adopted the mind-set of the slim – and is determined to keep it.

Keep an eye out for habits!

If you've made it this far, you, like Beth, will have adopted a slim mind-set. But bad habits are sneaky little pests. They'll crawl back into your life without you noticing, if you let them. Phase Five is designed to prevent this. It's a simple collection of tools that you can use in your daily life to prevent the reappearance of your old negative habitweb. Very quickly you'll naturally start using these tools without realising you're doing so.

Phase Five differs slightly to the previous four phases of the *No Diet Diet*. It's not a day-by-day (or step-by-step) programme. Instead, it contains a series of simple tasks that you need to do from time to time. Some should ideally be done each day. Others around once a month. The actual frequency is not critical. If you skip a day – or even a week – there's no need to worry. But do try and do the tasks at the recommended frequencies.

In the first instance, it might be an idea to keep a diary or calendar handy to remind yourself to use the habit-breaking tools. This will also allow you to keep track of how often you've used them. Please remember that the aim is to embed habit-breaking into your daily life. If you perform the tasks regularly and consistently, you'll be certain to maintain your weight loss and continue slimming down to your ideal weight. And the more you practise, the better you'll become.

Briefly, Phase Five asks you to:

•   **Keep an eye out for emerging bad habits using the *No Diet Diet* habit-spotter. This should be done every month or so.**

•   **Continue breaking bad habits by constantly – and subtly – enhancing your mental and behavioural flexibility. You should aim to do this every day.**

- **Carry on enhancing your personality in such crucial areas as awareness and balance. Again, this is something you should aim to do every day.**

Daily tasks

Thinking is the habit-slayer-in-chief. If you actively think about what you're doing – whatever it is – then bad habits can't sneak back into your life and seize control. So each day we'd like you to:

- **Think for a short while about a different thought-dimension, such as conscience or fearlessness. We did something similar in Phase Four.**

- **Explore different personality areas, such as assertive–unassertive or calm/relaxed–energetic/driven. We did something similar in Phase Two.**

Thought-dimensions

From now on, each day we'd like you to think carefully for a few minutes about a different *thought-dimension,* such as awareness or fearlessness. A thought-dimension is simply a way of thinking. For example, balance and self-responsibility are both thought-dimensions. We'd then like you to apply this thought-dimension to the way you react to people and situations. To refresh your mind about this concept, it might be worth re-reading the introduction to Phase Four.

At this point you might be feeling a little daunted. In Phase Four you applied each thought-dimension to a specific person and situation. That may appear far easier than applying it throughout the whole day. Don't worry. Obviously we'd like you to apply these dimensions flawlessly, but we realise that you – like us – are not perfect. There are times when you will not succeed. It's important to remember that it's the attempt that counts. Every time you make the attempt, even if you 'fail', you will improve. The aim is not to be a saint but to make steady progress. You should also not become obsessive about it. Every step you take from now on ensures that you'll embed your newly discovered slim mind-set, even if you fail to act perfectly throughout the whole day. And that is what will ensure that you stay slim forever.

The five thought-dimensions we'd like you to apply are:

1.   **Awareness**: of the environment, of yourself and the results of your thoughts and actions.

2.   **Self-responsibility**: accepting personal accountability for yourself, your decisions and your life, however difficult the situation.

3.   **Balance**: balancing the effort you put in to the importance of the task at hand.

4.   **Fearlessness**: never making decisions or behaving out of fear.

5.   **Conscience**: taking account of what you believe is right and moral, and then acting on it.

If you'd like some more guidance, why not refer back to Phase Four or have a look at Chapter Four: The Science of *Doing Something Different*.

We get the best out of life when our thoughts and behaviour are guided by these five thought-dimensions (they are also called the 'constancies' in FIT Science). Ideally, you'd always behave flexibly, with good conscience, total awareness, self-responsibility and fearlessness while making sure that life remains in balance. That's the ideal. Phase Five aims to move you towards this goal. You'll achieve this by:

Each day choosing a thought-dimension and applying it when the appropriate opportunities arise.

Exploring your personality

Each day we'd also like you to keep habits at bay by exploring and enhancing different facets of your personality. If you cast your mind back to Phase Two, you'll remember that each day you began pushing back the frontiers of your character. It might be worth re-reading that section to refresh your mind about the concept. The idea was to expand your behavioural flexibility. For example, if you are normally introverted, we asked you to behave more like an extrovert. Each day in Phase Five we'd like you to do something similar.

The parts of your personality you should explore are the same as those in Phase Two:

- **Assertive–Unassertive**

- **Calm/Relaxed–Energetic/Driven**

- **Definite–Flexible**

- **Spontaneous–Systematic**

- **Introverted–Extroverted**

- **Conventional–Unconventional**

- **Individual-centred–Group-centred**

These personality areas are known as behavioural-dimensions. We'd now like to measure these dimensions. Then we'd like to gauge how much your flexibility has improved over the past month or so. After that, we'll show you how to increase your behavioural flexibility even more. Our research shows that most people need to increase their flexibility a little further if they are to embed their habit-breaking ways permanently.

Rating your behavioural flexibility

Look at the list of seven behavioural-dimensions below then rate yourself out of ten. For example, if you are capable of being both extremely assertive and extremely unassertive, as the situation requires, then your score should be the maximum of ten. If you feel that you can only ever behave in one way then your score should be one. Your behavioural flexibility score reflects your ability to tailor your behaviour to get the most out of life.

Then, for each dimension, you'll need to come up with three scores, one for before you started the programme, one for how you are now, and one for how you want to be. To do this, you'll just need to answer these three questions:

1.   How flexible were you at the start of the *No Diet Diet*? Ten represents maximum flexibility in all situations, whereas one signifies very little. Put this score in the Start column.

2.   How flexible are you now? Again, you should score yourself out of ten. Put this number in the Now column.

3.   What is your goal? Is it ten, or perhaps less? Be realistic, but also remember that to achieve your potential you may need to stretch yourself a little. Put this score in the Goal column.

		Start	Now	Goal
Unassertive	Assertive	————	————	————
Calm/Relaxed	Energetic/Driven	————	————	————
Definite	Flexible	————	————	————
Spontaneous	Systematic	————	————	————
Introverted	Extroverted	————	————	————
Conventional	Unconventional	————	————	————
Individual-centred	Group-centred	————	————	————
Total		————	————	————

Add up your scores for each column and enter these in the Total boxes.

To enhance your flexibility, you'll need to increase your Now score towards ten for each dimension. We want you to set a high goal for yourself. If your Goal is much less than ten for each dimension (and your overall total much less than 70) you should ask yourself why you're not stretching yourself more.

Increasing your behavioural flexibility

To increase your score, you'll need to increase the range of behaviours you feel comfortable with. As you can no doubt guess, you'll achieve this by *Doing Something Different*. Each day you need to try to expand your behavioural range by acting differently with a person and reacting differently (but appropriately) to a situation.

Acting differently with a person

Choose someone. It could be a friend, colleague or even someone you dislike intensely. The choice is yours. You should then act differently towards them when the situation requires it. Alternatively, if your relationship with someone is in a rut, or you are involved in a conflict or a 'personality clash', this could be a good time to try a different approach. It might be worth re-reading pages 92–119 of Phase Two to give yourself some ideas about the ways in which you can alter your behaviour. Remember, in the long run, your aim is to enhance your flexibility with everyone. So although initially you might focus your attention on one particular person, over time you should try and enhance your flexibility with everyone.

Reacting differently to a situation

Now choose a situation. It could be one which causes you stress, makes you angry, induces frustration or perhaps makes you very happy and contented. Again, the choice is yours. You should now aim to behave differently to how you would normally. Your goal is to maximise your flexibility in order to maximise the benefit to you. The aim is to make the most of situations rather than just reacting out of habit. It might be worth re-reading pages 94–120 of Phase Two to give yourself some ideas about the ways in which you can alter your behaviour. Initially, you may choose to focus your efforts on one particular situation, but your long-term aim should be to maximise your flexibility all of the time. And remember, act for the best, not out of habit!

Never, Ever Give Up

If you follow the *No Diet Diet* then, according to our research, you're virtually guaranteed to lose a satisfying amount of weight. But if your weight loss has stalled, or is less than you hoped for, don't despair. Here are the causes – and the solutions.

Your initial weight loss isn't dramatic

The *No Diet Diet* is a slow burn. It takes time to lose weight. If you've given up because your progress was less than you hoped for, then please have another go. In the long run we don't believe you'll be disappointed. We've studied over 1,000 people as part of our research. Our clients lose between 1–2 lb (0.5–1 kg) per week. But this average covers quite a wide range. Many of our clients lose more than the average, whereas a few manage to lose 'only' 3 lb (1.5 kg) per month. However, if you extrapolate this over three or six months, then this amounts to an awful lot of weight. People spend years yo-yo dieting. So even if you've 'only' lost a little weight during the initial 28-step programme, then you're already ahead of the people who are still yo-yo dieting.

You're not behaving sufficiently differently

Occasionally, people following the *No Diet Diet* find it difficult to move outside their comfort zone. This is understandable. Your habits are cosy, warm and comfortable, so it can be diffi-cult to leave their shelter behind. Our programme is based upon making small, progressive changes on a step-by-step basis. It's not what you do that counts – or even the degree to which you change – it's the process of *Doing Something Different* that ensures you lose weight. Having said that, you

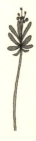

have to leave your comfort zone. If you feel a frisson of excitement, slight uneasiness or just a bit nervous, then you've probably got it about right. To succeed, you do not have to terrify yourself or make big, bold leaps in the dark, you simply have to take small, progressive steps forward. These changes are essential for habit-breaking. If you succeed, then you will lose weight. So moving outside your comfort zone is essential.

Like most things in life, you get out of the *No Diet Diet* what you put in. And whatever way you look at it, the programme is easier than calorie or carb counting, ploughing through GI and GL tables, or suffering the anxiety and depression associated with food diets. So please carry on with the programme.

You worry about what people will think

Many 'non-dieters' are initially worried about other people's reactions when they begin the programme and start behaving differently. This can be a big block to your progress. Many of our habits and behaviours are partly kept in place by other people. They expect us to behave in the same old ways, so we do. Don't let that attitude stop you from trying new things. Why not try getting them on your side? Talk to them about the programme and what you hope to achieve. Why not explain to them that this is the best chance you have to get what you want? Once they realise that the *No Diet Diet* will help you lose weight and become happier and healthier, we're sure that they'll begin supporting you. You never know, they might even want to try it themselves. So why not encourage your friends and family to follow the *No Diet Diet* too? You'll get far more out of the programme if you do it with others. And while you're at it, why not set up a *No Diet Diet* club of your own too?

To recap

- **Each day choose both a different person and a situation, and behave differently.**

- **Every month you should re-assess your behavioural flexibility scores. Why not put it into your diary now?**

Monthly tasks

The most important thing you can do each month to stay slim is to habit-spot. Bad habits have a nasty way of creeping back inside you. If you've completed the first four phases of the *No Diet Diet*, it will take many months for the negative habitweb to re-establish itself. But your habits will come crawling back unless you keep watching out for them. You can never eliminate all of your habits (and remember some do have benefits too), the aim is simply to ensure that they don't control your life. So as soon as you notice a habit, it's best to break it there and then. When they're young they're still vulnerable and easy to finish off. The longer you leave it, the tougher they'll become.

To keep on top of them, you should work through the habit-spotter on page 218 every month. It should only take you a few minutes. Spotting your own habits can sometimes be a little difficult. To get around this problem, it's a good idea to get someone else to help spot them for you. We've included an extra habit-spotter for a friend or partner to fill in. You'll probably find this very revealing indeed!

Preparing to habit-spot

Before you do your first round of habit-spotting you'll need to do a little preparation. You should only need to do this the once, but feel free to do it as many times as you wish. After all, the better you get at it, the more flexible you'll become and the more weight you'll lose.

The first thing you'll need to do is learn how to notice other people's habits. It's an awful lot easier (and more fun) to start off watching other people than it is to focus on yourself. You can easily spend hours looking out for other people's habits. And you can virtually guarantee that they won't be aware of them. You'll probably notice very quickly that there's a direct link between someone's habits and their weight. The more habit-bound they are, the more overweight they'll be! Pretty soon you'll be looking out for other people's habits every time you have a spare few moments.

You'll also notice that they fall into seven broad categories:

- **Thinking habits** These can be strong attitudes, biases, prejudices and reactions. Automatic thoughts, such as, 'He's got long hair and a pierced nose, so he must be weird', are examples of thinking habits that reflect a closed mind.

- **Habits of the past** A good example is automaticity, or always reacting and responding completely without thought. Bearing grudges, using the past to justify the present and repeating the same mistakes over and over again are all habits of the past. We know of one woman who still hasn't got over another girl turning up at school with an identical bag to hers – 25 years ago! So get over it and move on.

- **Relationship habits** These include the way you interact with people. For example, always being confrontational or passive instead of reacting in the most effective way possible is a relationship habit. Consistently having a high or low regard for others is one too. So, if you constantly nag another person and they don't do what you want, why not stop blaming them? It's time you stopped nagging and tried something different.

- **Strategy habits** These include rigidity, or always using the same or similar solutions to solve different problems. Strategy habits also include consistently putting off tasks until the last minute, or always passing on problems to other people instead of dealing with them yourself.

- **Ego habits** These include habits relating to power, status and territory. For example, bosses who insist that their staff refer to them by a certain title or executives who like to have their name on the door and a designated parking space are all showing that they're trapped by their ego habits. If you have habits that exist merely to demonstrate your power, or to mark your territory, it may be time to let go a little and *Do Something Different*.

- **Personal habits** These include idiosyncrasies, irritations and annoyances. We all notice when others have 'quirks of character', but are generally unaware of our own. You could try watching yourself on video. We know people who've done this and were stunned by how irritating their giggles were or shocked by how often they said 'you know'.

- **Perspective habits** These include the inability to prioritise, for example spending too much time on the detail and not enough on the most important tasks. Irrational fears can also often arise from perspective habits. Feeling terrified that you'll make a fool of yourself comes from the irrational thought that everyone is watching you – they're not!

Spotting habits in other people

You should now spend a little time looking out for other people's habits. They will probably all fall into one of the categories we've just outlined. Wherever you find people, you'll find habits. And each time you do a little habit-spotting, it will get easier to notice your own. It's quite addictive.

List the habits you've spotted in other people here:

Thinking habits

Who are you watching? _____

What have you noticed?

_____

_____

_____

_____

Habits of the past

Who are you watching? _____

What have you noticed?

_____

_____

_____

_____

Relationship habits

Who are you watching? _____

What have you noticed?

_____

_____

_____

_____

Strategy habits

Who are you watching? _____

What have you noticed?

_____

_____

_____

_____

Ego habits

Who are you watching? _____

What have you noticed?

_____

_____

_____

_____

Personal habits

Who are you watching? _____

What have you noticed?

_____

_____

_____

_____

Perspective habits

Who are you watching? _____

What have you noticed?

_____

_____

_____

_____

Remember, you only need to do this preparation once, but feel free to do it as many times as you wish.

Spotting your own habits

After spending a little time spotting habits in other people, you're now ready to turn the spotlight on yourself. Several habits should be quite obvious. You know that you have them. Now's the time to face up to them and tackle them!

A number of habits, however, are unconscious and buried deeper. To help bring these to your attention, we've developed the *No Diet Diet* 'habit-spotter'. You'll find this over the page. Try to be as honest as you can when you answer the habit-spotter questions. If you don't face up to your habits, you won't be able to tackle them effectively.

Often it's easier for others to spot your more ingrained habits. Friends, family and colleagues will notice things about you that have passed you by for years. So, after you've filled in the first habit-spotter on the next page, you should ask a close friend or partner to complete the second questionnaire, which follows on immediately from the first. If they are honest, they'll help you uncover the habits you didn't know you had. So encourage them to be ruthlessly candid!

The *No Diet Diet* habit-spotter: yourself

Answer the following questions as honestly as possible:

How often do you

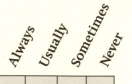

	Always	Usually	Sometimes	Never
Listen to others with empathy and understanding?				
Do something that's bad for you?				
Change where you sit at mealtimes?				
Say things without thinking?				
Have a go at something you're not very good at?				
Sit in the same place to watch TV?				
Try to learn something new?				
Wear the same style of clothes?				
Try a new place to go out for a drink or a meal?				
Dismiss other people's ideas or suggestions?				
Suggest ways to make life more interesting?				
Say that life is boring?				

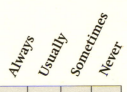

	Always	Usually	Sometimes	Never
Think about thinking?				
Have the same things for breakfast?				
Look for new challenges in your life?				
Express the same opinion repeatedly?				
Change the newspaper they read?				
Watch a regularly scheduled TV programme?				
Do something that surprises those around you?				
Buy things from the same shops?				
Find it easy to forget negative things people have done to you in the past?				
Revisit the same holiday destination?				
Change the circle of friends you mix with?				
Do the same things on the same days or the same evenings?				
Try to meet people who challenge and inspire you?				

The *No Diet Diet* habit-spotter: other

Now ask someone who knows you well to answer the following questions. Tell them to be honest ...

Answer these questions about _____ (name)

How often does this person

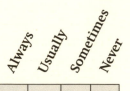

	Always	Usually	Sometimes	Never
Listen to others with empathy and understanding?				
Do something that's bad for them?				
Change where they sit at mealtimes?				
Say things without thinking?				
Have a go at something they're not very good at?				
Sit in the same place to watch TV?				
Try to learn something new?				
Wear the same style of clothes?				
Try a new place to go out for a drink or a meal?				
Dismiss other people's ideas or suggestions?				
Suggest ways to make life more interesting?				

	Always	Usually	Sometimes	Never
Say that life is boring?				
Think about thinking?				
Have the same things for breakfast?				
Look for new challenges in their life?				
Express the same opinion repeatedly?				
Change the newspaper they read?				
Watch a regularly scheduled TV programme?				
Do something that surprises those around them?				
Buy things from the same shops?				
Find it easy to forget negative things people have done to them in the past?				
Revisit the same holiday destination?				
Change the circle of friends they mix with?				
Do the same things on the same days or the same evenings?				
Try to meet people who challenge and inspire them?				

Scoring

Habits spotted by yourself

Scoring the habit-spotter is not as complex as it first appears. You will see that there are shaded and non-shaded items on the habit-spotter.

- **The questions in the non-shaded boxes highlight *negative habits*.**

- **The questions in the shaded boxes highlight *positive habits*.**

Score the negative (non-shaded) items out of three. That is:

   0   for 'Never'   **2**   for 'Usually'
   1   for 'Sometimes'   **3**   for 'Always'

Now add up these scores, which should give you a value between 0 and 36.

Write your total score for negative habits here: _____

Now you need to score the positive, or shaded, boxes. Also score these on a scale from 0 to 3. That is:

   3   for 'Never'   **1**   for 'Usually'
   2   for 'Sometimes'   **0**   for 'Always'

Now add up these scores, which should give you a value between 0 and 39.

Write your total score for positive habits here: _____

Now add both the negative and positive (non-shaded and shaded) scores together.

Write your total score here: _____

How did you do?

The higher your total score, the more habitual you are. So, if you scored:

Between 0 and 25

This is good! You don't have many negative habits and the habits that you do have are mostly positive ones. We hope that you've reached this happy state as a result of doing the *No Diet Diet*. We also hope that you'll continue using our daily and monthly habit-breaking tools. Our guess is that you'll have lost more weight than average, too.

Between 26 and 50

You're on the borderline and need to do some careful self-monitoring. You have a few too many bad habits and not enough good ones. If you don't shake off some of those bad habits then you'll find that you won't lose much more excess weight. So please keep following the principles in this book and you'll be well on the way to being less habit-bound – and to weighing even less.

Between 51 and 75

You are a human habit-machine and need to do something quickly! If you've followed the programme in this book then we doubt that you've genuinely scored so high. So our guess is that you've done the habit-spotter before doing the programme. That's fine, you've proved one thing; you urgently need to do the *Do Something Different* programme.

If, however, you have completed phases one to four, then we recommend that you re-do the programme. We doubt that you'll have lost much weight in any case. The amount of weight you lose on our programme relates to how many bad habits you break. Re-doing the programme will ease you further along the weight-loss path. Please remember, you haven't failed, you've discovered something very profound about yourself. Now you can put this new-found knowledge to great use. So please re-do our programme and you'll be amazed at how much weight you'll lose.

Habits spotted by a friend, partner or relation

Again, you will see that there are positive and negative items in the habit-spotter.

• **The questions in the non-shaded boxes highlight *negative habits*.**

• **The questions in the shaded boxes highlight *positive habits*.**

Now you need to score your answers. Score the negative (non-shaded) items from 0 to 3. That is:

0 for 'Never'   **2** for 'Usually'
1 for 'Sometimes'   **3** for 'Always'

Now add up these scores, which should give you a value between 0 and 36.

Write your total score for negative habits here: _____

Now you need to score the positive or shaded boxes. Also score these on a scale from 0 to 3. That is:

3 for 'Never'   **1** for 'Usually'
2 for 'Sometimes'   **0** for 'Always'

Now add up these scores, which should give you a value between 0 and 39.

Write your total score for positive habits here: _____

Now add both the negative and positive (non-shaded and shaded) scores together.

Write your total score here: _____

Comparing notes

This is where habit-spotting gets even more interesting. There's probably a difference in scores between the habit-spotter you did and the one completed by your friend, partner or family member. These scores will vary depending on how good you are at noticing your own habits. You should now compare these two overall scores, and what they mean, so please refer back to 'How did you do?' on page 223. Doing so will give you a good idea where your 'hidden' habits lie and the areas on which you need to focus your attention. Please remember that one of the most important steps you can take towards breaking a habit is noticing that you've got it in the first place. Once you've done this, it's often a relatively small step to break it.

For example, if you notice that you always watch the same TV programmes, read the same newspaper, eat dinner in the same seat and go on holiday to the same place, you know what you have to do, don't you?

❀ Moving forward

Now you need to list the habits highlighted by the habit-spotter (space is provided for you to do this on page 225). You should then spend a few minutes thinking about how you're going to break these habits and the steps you'll need to take to achieve this.

You also need to write down the habits that were highlighted by your friend, partner or family member, and which you didn't know you had (space is provided for you to do this on page 229). Once you've listed these, you can start thinking of ways of breaking these habits too. Remember, the idea is to take you out of your comfort zone. If you do this, you'll continue striding down the weight-loss road.

For each of your habits, you should also ask yourself the following questions to help focus your mind:

1. *Is the habit something you were born with?* Many people believe that they were born to be the way they are. They claim that genetics or upbringing made them the person they are today. In most cases, this is simply not true. Scientific research shows that we can choose to behave very differently to this 'natural tendency'. It's a matter of choosing to get the most out of life.

2. *Do you see the habit as an aspect of your personality?* You might have developed a personal style, but that doesn't mean that your 'style' or 'character' always dictates the best response to a person or situation. Your personality isn't fixed for life – it should be allowed to grow constantly and help you explore new ways of enjoying life. Remember, you can change for the better!

3. *Did you learn the habit?* You probably did learn this habit, but you may also have become used to misapplying it. Much

of the time the habit probably works against you rather than for you. If you learnt it, you can also unlearn it.

4.   *Is it a habit you've adopted from someone in your family or from a friend or colleague?* People often pick up habits from other people. But what's right for other people may not be right for you.

5.   *Are you good at the habit?* People tend to stick to what they know best and become experts at defending the way they are. They claim that it's part of their personality or character. But that doesn't make the habit right for them or the best solution to all of their problems.

6.   *Is the habit good for you generally?* Some habits are undoubtedly useful, but many others are not. So you should ask this question of all of your habits, and make a sensible, rational decision.

7.   *Will the habit be good for you in the future?* Just because it worked for you in the past doesn't mean it will be right for you in the future. Keep a constant lookout for all of your habits and reassess their usefulness regularly.

8.   *What are the advantages of breaking this habit?* There will always be advantages to breaking a habit. If you are not constantly reassessing them, the chances are you have an ingrained problem.

9.   *Do you want to change the habit? If not, why not?* You should have very good reasons for putting up with a habit. If you do decide to stick with it, make sure it's for a solid reason and not just because it's easier that way.

10.   *How will you make the change if you do decide to get rid of this habit?* Use the *Do Something Different* approach!

Final thoughts

Have you reassessed your behavioural flexibility scores? Why not put next month's reassessment into your diary now? And while you're at it, why not put a reminder in to re-run the habit-spotter too?

What new habits have you noticed in yourself and how do you plan to break them?

What habits were noticed by the other person and how do you plan to break them?

_____

_____

_____

_____

_____

_____

_____

_____

_____

_____

_____

_____

_____

_____

_____

_____

_____

_____

KEY POINTS

- You will continue losing around 2 lb (1 kg) per week until your ideal figure emerges. You'll achieve this because you've adopted a slim mind-set.

- If you allow your bad habits to sneak back into your life, you are likely to start gaining weight again.

- Phase Five is designed to embed habit-breaking and weight loss into your daily life. It is a collection of tools to help achieve this. Some should ideally be used each day. Others once a month.

- If you don't manage to use the habit-breaking tools for a while, don't worry. But don't leave it too long. Bad habits constantly try and creep back into your life. As soon as you stop breaking them, they'll begin imprisoning you again.

- Keep a diary or calendar on hand to remind yourself to use the habit-breaking tools.

CHAPTER ELEVEN

Doing Something Different for Life

Habit, if not resisted, soon becomes necessity.

St Augustine

By now you'll have realised that we're evangelists, not only for a radically new way of losing weight, but also for helping people change their lives for the better. We hope that you now understand why we've been so relentlessly positive throughout this book. The *Do Something Different* approach opens up whole new vistas for people to explore and radically improve their lives.

A way of living

You undoubtedly did the *No Diet Diet* to lose weight – no more, no less – and this is what you've achieved. But just pause for a moment and reflect on all of the other benefits arising from the *No Diet Diet*. The *No Diet Diet* is much *much* more than a diet, it's a way of life. People who follow the programme tend to be more successful. Their relationships are more harmonious. They are happier and more contented. In many ways this is just common sense. The more adaptable you are – and the greater your range of behaviours – the more quickly you can take advantage of new situations. This leads to greater financial and personal success.

It also means you find new situations less stressful. In turn, of course, this ensures that you are a more grounded and secure person. Personal and financial security helps you become happier and more contented. It's a virtuous circle.

By now you'll have lost a significant amount of weight. And this weight loss should continue for many more weeks and months. In fact, if you continue habit-spotting and doing things differently, you'll slim down to your body's natural weight and maintain it for the rest of your life. Constantly exploring all that life has to offer is the secret to achieving permanent weight loss. After all, that is how the slim maintain their weight. They are not 'naturally' thin. They don't have a different metabolism to you. Their genes are no better or worse than yours. They are simply slim because they are mentally flexible and chip away at their habitwebs. Never forget this.

The secret to remaining slim is to live life a little differently each day. Live it to the full. Big changes aren't required. Remaining flexible involves making small, progressive changes. It means pausing on your way to work and watching the world go by. It also means rearranging the furniture, buying a different magazine or sitting somewhere new. It means savouring the smell of freshly cut grass in the park, listening to the different layers of music in your favourite song, changing your radio station or making a list of your childhood dreams. Whatever you do today, ask yourself whether you can do it differently. Subtly alter your character from day to day; be assertive, be passive, be different ... This is the secret to remaining slim.

We hope that you've enjoyed doing the *No Diet Diet*. If you have, please tell your friends and family about it. Your voice can help others abandon yo-yo dieting, lose weight and become 'non-dieters'. In time, they may come to realise that living life to the full is so much more important than dieting.

And if you're ever in any doubt about anything, *Do Something Different*!

Appendix:
Frequently Asked Questions

The programme is different to any diet I've been on before (and I've tried them all). How can switching off the TV or singing in the bath help me lose weight?

It does seem a little odd at first, but once you understand the science behind the *No Diet Diet* it becomes far clearer. Why not re-read Chapters Two and Four to gain a deeper understanding? The *No Diet Diet* is based on many years of scientific research. It shows clearly that the more you chip away at your habitweb by behaving differently, the more weight you'll lose.

I'm seriously overweight. Can I still use the programme?

Yes! It's a healthy programme that should benefit everyone, unlike food- and exercise-based diets. If you have any doubts, check with your GP.

Do I have to do everything in the order specified in the book?

The different phases of the *No Diet Diet* are carefully designed to help you break your bad habits in a gradual and progressive way. So you should do Phases One to Four in the order they're given. However, you can do the steps within each of the phases in a different order. For example, there might be a day when it's difficult for you to do a certain step, so rather than not doing it at all, you can swap it with another from within the same phase. Having said that, we can see very few reasons – or excuses – to deviate from the book.

If I fall off the wagon and have a bad habit day, do I have to go back to the beginning of the programme?

No. If you do miss a day, just pick up from where you left off.

I get stuck on some of the tasks and can't think of anything new to do. Help!

Why not try buddying up with a friend so that you can exchange ideas and support each other? You could also try altering your mental perspective. Think of what you normally do then STOP. Often you'll find that simply stopping and observing the task in your mind will give you some new leads. You could also try shifting your mental focus in and out so that you see either the bigger picture – or just one part of the task. As soon as you shift your focus you'll naturally see many different ways of tackling the problem.

Some days I just don't have the motivation to stick with the programme. Will I fail?

It's only natural for motivation to wane from time to time. Following the *No Diet Diet* is no different. It's important to remember that you won't fail the *No Diet Diet*. But some people find it takes them a little longer to get what they want. If this happens to you, try taking smaller steps forward. There's no rush. Each day, if you do things a little differently, you'll lose weight. Your enthusiasm will soon return, and when it does, you'll feel more confident about taking bigger steps forward.

Should I be on a low-calorie diet at the same time?

You can't lose weight unless the amount of energy you burn up exceeds the amount you consume. If you follow the *No Diet Diet* you'll find that you naturally start eating more healthily and leading a more active life. The *No Diet Diet* helps you break the habits that have stopped you from doing this in the past. And you'll be surprised by the results.

Do I need to take more exercise to lose weight on the *No Diet Diet*?

It's certainly a good idea to exercise regularly. It's a key part of living a long, healthy and happy life. Although you're not required to take exercise on the *No Diet Diet*, you'll probably find that you naturally start leading a more active life. Some of the habit-breaking tasks in the *No Diet Diet* may also help you become more active, but that's not their primary aim. They are simply designed to help you break free from your unhealthy habits.

I've lost quite a few pounds, but my weight has plateaued – what am I doing wrong?

We're all individuals. Everyone differs in their natural rate of weight loss. Some people lose weight rapidly, others slowly, or in stages interspersed with plateaus. It's important to remember that the *No Diet Diet* can be a slow burn. It can take time to lose weight. If you're considering giving up because your progress is less than you hoped for, please don't. In the long run you won't be disappointed. We've studied over 1,000 people as part of our university research. Our clients lose between 1 lb and 2 lb (0.5 kg and 1 kg) per week. But this average covers quite a wide range. Many of our clients lose more than the average whereas a few manage to lose 'only' 3 lb (1.5 kg) per month. However, if you extrapolate this over three or six months, then this amounts to an awful lot of weight. People spend years yo-yo dieting. So even if you've 'only' lost a few pounds during the initial 28-step programme, then you're already ahead of the people who are still yo-yo dieting.

It's been two weeks and I haven't lost any weight yet. If I went on a crash diet I'd be slimmer by now. Why should I carry on?

You probably would lose weight more rapidly on a crash diet, but how long would it last? Around 95 per cent of people who go on a diet weigh the same or more a year later. Is that what you want? If you follow the *No Diet Diet* the weight loss is permanent. Diets are also bad for your mental and physical health. We suggest that you re-read Chapter Three if you're seriously considering a food diet.

A few people experience slow weight loss when they follow the *No Diet Diet*. Generally speaking, the more habits you break – and the more flexible you become – the more weight you'll lose. So if you're not losing any weight (or very little) you should try making bigger changes in your life. Are you persistently choosing the easiest options in the programme rather than the ones that take you outside your comfort zone? This could be the root cause of the problem. Like most things in life, you get out of the *No Diet Diet* what you put in. And whatever way you look at it, the programme is easier than calorie or carb counting, ploughing through GI and GL tables, or suffering the anxiety and depression associated with food diets. Please remember that you won't fail the *No Diet Diet*, but your progress may be slower than average. And, what the hell, slow weight loss is healthy weight loss!

My friends also want to do the *No Diet Diet*. Can we do it together or should we do it alone?

It's great to work with other people on the programme. That way, you can share your experiences, support each other, and enjoy new activities together.

Can my 13-year-old daughter go on the *No Diet Diet*?

The *No Diet Diet* will certainly be better for her than a food diet. If she's seriously considering a diet then she should read Chapter Three, which highlights all of the problems and failings of diets. We'd also caution you against feeding your daughter's fears about her weight. If she is not overweight, perhaps you should be reassuring her about her body instead. If she's only slightly overweight, you could try encouraging her to become more behaviourally flexible without actually putting her on the *No Diet Diet*. That way, she'll get the benefits of the programme without having any of her fears about her weight inadvertently reinforced. If she does need to lose a significant amount of weight then she'll have a good headstart on the rest of us. Young people tend to be relatively flexible and not overly habit-bound. For her, the *No Diet Diet* should be even easier and more fun to do. To encourage her, you could try being a positive role model by following the *No Diet Diet* yourself. That way, you'll gain all of the benefits of the programme too.

I'm quite an anxious person and I actually like things to stay the way they are. Is it normal to worry about making changes?

Of course it's natural to feel a bit anxious when you start moving outside your 'comfort zone'. After all, that's what the comfort zone is – it's comfortable – so you won't want to leave it. Our clinical trials have discovered that anxiety and fear are reduced by the *No Diet Diet*. It's a side effect we're quite happy about – it's certainly better than smelly breath and food cravings! If you're naturally anxious, start off by making smaller changes in your life. Don't be over-ambitious. You can also try making some of the changes in private at first. If introduced gradually, small changes in your daily routine needn't be overwhelming and nobody need know you're doing them.

I'm going on holiday and it will be difficult to stick to the
***No Diet Diet*. Should I leave it until I get back?**

A holiday is the perfect time to do things differently! Don't see it
as a break in the programme – carry on regardless. A holiday is a
great time to reflect on your habits and the rut you've found
yourself in. While you're away try not to slip into your usual holiday habits, such as eating the same food or visiting the same
bars. Try and make this holiday a little different.

My family don't like some of the tasks I have to do on the
***No Diet Diet*, what can I do about it?**

Many 'non-dieters' are initially worried about other people's reactions when they begin the programme and start behaving differently. This can be a big block on progress. Many of our habits and
behaviours are partly kept in place by other people. They expect
us to behave in the same old ways, so we do. Don't let that attitude
stop you from trying new things. Instead, why not try getting
them on your side? Talk to them about the programme and what
you hope to achieve. Why not explain to them that this is the best
chance you have to get what you want? Once they realise that the
No Diet Diet will help you lose weight and become happier and
healthier, they'll probably begin supporting you. And you never
know, they might even want to try it as well! So why not encourage your friends and family to follow the No Diet Diet too? You'll get
far more out of the programme if you do it with others. And while
you're at it, why not set up a No Diet Diet club of your own too?

It's important for me to follow my religious beliefs. Can I do
the *No Diet Diet* without compromising them?

Yes! We're not suggesting that you try anything that runs against
your beliefs. Nor are we advocating anything that could harm
you or anyone else. We've found that people can easily follow the
No Diet Diet without compromising their moral or religious principles.

I find it difficult to understand some of the ideas in the *No Diet Diet*. Am I just not clever enough to follow the programme?

Not at all. You were clever enough to buy this book! We've tried to make some rather complex psychological theories as straightforward as possible. If we have failed, then we can only apologise. It's important to remember that you don't need to understand the science behind the *No Diet Diet* to lose weight. We've explained the psychology of *Doing Something Different* at various points in this book for the people who want to understand it. If you're not interested but still want to lose weight then all you have to do is follow the programme. If you're ever confused about the terms we use, you can always refer to the Glossary on page 243.

People say I'm slim, but I feel fat. Can I still use the plan to lose weight?

If your Body Mass Index is between 18.5 and 25 then you are already a healthy weight. The BMI is a standard measure of body weight relative to height. You can find BMI charts on the Internet, in doctor's surgeries, or you can calculate it yourself easily enough. It is simply your weight in kilograms divided by your height in metres squared (i.e. multiplied by itself). People who've dieted a lot can begin seeing themselves as fatter than they actually are. This can be a sign of 'body dysmorphia' and may be linked to an eating disorder. If you're worried about this then you should seek professional help. Start by talking to your GP about it. Having said that, as society becomes fatter, what is considered a 'normal' weight is slowly increasing. A plump person from 30 years ago is more likely to be considered a normal weight today. This is why you should stick to the medical definition of 'normal', which is a Body Mass Index of 18.5–25.

One of the best things about the *No Diet Diet* is that people naturally gravitate towards their ideal weight. So if you're truly overweight then you'll gradually lose your excess pounds. If, however, you're about right then you'll naturally maintain this weight.

How can I keep motivated after finishing the programme?

Virtually everyone who completes the initial 28-step programme becomes so inspired by the *No Diet Diet* that they naturally carry on breaking their habits. But if your enthusiasm does begin to wane then you should use the habit-breaking and monitoring tools detailed in Phase Five more often. You could also try re-doing some of the exercises in Phases One to Four. For example, you could try doing some of the weekly tasks outlined in Phases One and Three. Choose ones that are different to those you tried the first time around. And remember, the key to losing weight – and keeping it off permanently – is to break your habits by doing things differently.

I'm reaching the end of the *No Diet Diet*, where do I go next?

The *Do Something Different* programme isn't something that you should do for only a few weeks. We hope it becomes a philosophy that you follow for the rest of your life. That way, the pounds will stay off for good. Keep applying the ideas behind it and move forward. Don't just dream – do it!

Will I really carry on losing weight after I've finished the programme?

Yes!

Glossary of FIT Science Dimensions

Assertive: insisting upon your rights, or asking for what you want.

Awareness: the degree to which an individual monitors and attends to their internal and external worlds.

Balance: making sure each aspect of life receives due care and attention. The important parts should have a sufficient level of effort put into them and the person receive sufficient satisfaction from them.

Behave as expected: doing as others would normally expect you to.

Behave as wish: doing as you want to, not as others want you to.

Calm/Relaxed: being peaceful and not stressed; without tension.

Cautious: not trusting; being wary; concerned about risks.

Conscience: differentiating right from wrong and doing what is right.

Conventional: traditional, formal, according to normal custom.

Definite: certain, sure.

Emotional intelligence: recognising the emotions that you and others have and how to make them work for you, not against you.

Energetic/Driven: enthusiastic, motivated.

Extroverted: outgoing, sociable.

Fearlessness: acting without fear or trepidation; facing the unknown with the same bravado as the known.

Firm: resolute, standing by what you think, determined.

Flexible: open to change, willing and able to adapt.

Gentle: mild, kindly, subtle.

Group-centred: taking a team view, going along with the group.

Individual-centred: doing your own thing.

Introverted: inward-looking, not outgoing.

Lively: bubbly, effusive, full of life, animated.

Not lively: apparently lacking energy, laid-back.

Open-minded: open to new things, unprejudiced.

Predictable: habitual; people know what you will do next.

Proactive: taking the initiative, foreseeing and acting in advance.

Reactive: responding automatically, triggering actions.

Risky: taking risks, acting without due regard for consequences.

Self-responsibility: the degree to which a person accepts personal accountability for their world, irrespective of the impact of factors outside themselves. Self-responsibility is the motivator, self-limiter and mission-setter of a person.

Single-minded: very focused, knowing what and how.

Social intelligence: contributing in a positive way to people and society. It is making a difference for others, adding to the social capital of society in a selfless way.

Spontaneous: doing things on the spur of the moment.

Systematic: planning and considering in advance, orderly.

Trusting: believing that others are truthful and reliable.

Unassertive: not putting yourself forward, or asking for what you want.

Unconventional: different, willing to stand out.

Unpredictable: others not knowing what you will do next.

Wary: watchful or cautious, not readily trusting others.

Find out more – go to **www.nodietdietway.com** or **www.HabitDoctors.com**